Health Care in Transition

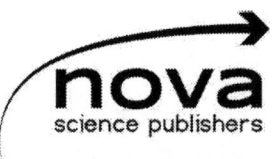

Health Care in Transition

Mobile Health: Advances in Research and Applications – Volume II
Gaurav Gupta, PhD, Varun Jaiswal, PhD, Manju Khari, PhD
and Nagesh Kumar, PhD (Editors)
2022. ISBN: 978-1-68507-988-8 (Hardcover)
2022. ISBN: 979-8-88697-247-4 (eBook)

Novel Perspectives in Economics of Personalized Medicine and Healthcare Systems
Marinko Škare, PhD, Romina Pržiklas Družeta, PhD,
Sandra Kraljević Pavelić, PhD (Editors)
2021. ISBN: 978-1-68507-390-9 (Hardcover)
2021. ISBN: 978-1-68507-393-0 (eBook)

Driving Hospitals Towards Performance: Practical Managerial Guidance to Reach the "Perfect Symphony"
Irene Gabutti, PhD (Author)
2021. ISBN: 978-1-68507-225-4 (Softcover)
2021. ISBN: 978-1-68507-382-4 (eBook)

Blockchain and Health: Transformation of Care and Impact of Digitalization
Jan Veuger, PhD (Editor)
2021. ISBN: 978-1-68507-232-2 (Hardcover)
2021. ISBN: 978-1-68507-260-5 (eBook)

Environmental Health in Malaysia
Hisham Atan Edinur, PhD, Mohd Tajuddin Abdullah, PhD and
Sabreena Safuan, PhD (Editors)
2021. ISBN: 978-1-68507-114-1 (Hardcover)
2021. ISBN: 978-1-68507-136-3 (eBook)

More information about this series can be found at
https://novapublishers.com/product-category/series/health-care-in-transition/

John Geyman, MD

The Future of U.S. Health Care?

Corporate Power vs. the Common Good

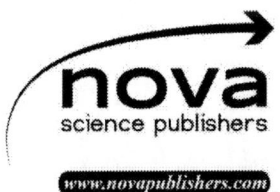

Copyright © 2022 by Nova Science Publishers, Inc.
https://doi.org/10.52305/SGHB6950

All rights reserved. No part of this book may be reproduced, stored in a retrieval system or transmitted in any form or by any means: electronic, electrostatic, magnetic, tape, mechanical photocopying, recording or otherwise without the written permission of the Publisher.

We have partnered with Copyright Clearance Center to make it easy for you to obtain permissions to reuse content from this publication. Simply navigate to this publication's page on Nova's website and locate the "Get Permission" button below the title description. This button is linked directly to the title's permission page on copyright.com. Alternatively, you can visit copyright.com and search by title, ISBN, or ISSN.

For further questions about using the service on copyright.com, please contact:
Copyright Clearance Center
Phone: +1-(978) 750-8400   Fax: +1-(978) 750-4470   E-mail: info@copyright.com

NOTICE TO THE READER

The Publisher has taken reasonable care in the preparation of this book, but makes no expressed or implied warranty of any kind and assumes no responsibility for any errors or omissions. No liability is assumed for incidental or consequential damages in connection with or arising out of information contained in this book. The Publisher shall not be liable for any special, consequential, or exemplary damages resulting, in whole or in part, from the readers' use of, or reliance upon, this material. Any parts of this book based on government reports are so indicated and copyright is claimed for those parts to the extent applicable to compilations of such works.

Independent verification should be sought for any data, advice or recommendations contained in this book. In addition, no responsibility is assumed by the Publisher for any injury and/or damage to persons or property arising from any methods, products, instructions, ideas or otherwise contained in this publication.

This publication is designed to provide accurate and authoritative information with regard to the subject matter covered herein. It is sold with the clear understanding that the Publisher is not engaged in rendering legal or any other professional services. If legal or any other expert assistance is required, the services of a competent person should be sought. FROM A DECLARATION OF PARTICIPANTS JOINTLY ADOPTED BY A COMMITTEE OF THE AMERICAN BAR ASSOCIATION AND A COMMITTEE OF PUBLISHERS.

Additional color graphics may be available in the e-book version of this book.

Library of Congress Cataloging-in-Publication Data

ISBN: 979-8-88697-338-9

Published by Nova Science Publishers, Inc. † New York

What a magnificent readable, graphical, pictorial handbook for people who want to replace the current wasteful, corrupt, hurtful and profit-at-any-cost healthcare industry with huge inputs of unlawful overbilling and misused government subsides. Dr. Geyman is the foremost public educator through annual books and pamphlets to arouse the citizenry regardless of political self-labels and turn Congress and the White House to passage of health insurance for all – single payer – having extensive efficiencies, life-saving and preventative advantages.

If you've ever felt anxiety, dread and fear while ill over your insurance coverage, "The Future of U.S. Health Care", is for you. The challenge is in this book's subtitle, "Corporate Power vs. The Common Good". Put this book in your library, send it to your members of Congress and demand a response and a meeting regarding the questions you want to put to them.

—Ralph Nader
June 13, 2022

This book is excellent. It's a nice, readable length, and its message is clear and strong. I think most readers will understand how health care should no longer be driven by the business ethic when the service ethic is in dire need of relief from intrusion by the business culture, so that we can place the patient first.

—Don McCanne, MD, family physician, Senior Health Policy Fellow and past President of Physicians for a National Health Program (PNHP), CA, USA

John Geyman is a grand master of organizing and presenting data on U. S. health system failings. He tells a clear, if sordid, tale of pervasive corporate infiltration of a system which should properly be guided by the imperative of clinical care for all. He bemoans how decades of corporate "consolidation brings with it more cost-sharing ... and reduced access across the board." He laments how corporate interests and their government allies promote medical advances based on market value, with little evidence of their value to patients. But he does not advocate caving to past trends and present dysfunction. He offers hope for transformation: "The current system is falling apart and is unsustainable ... public and political pressure will grow for reform." We can adopt the highly functional health coverage in all other wealthy countries. John's book should be in everyone's health care reform toolkit.

—Jim Kahn, MD, MPH, Professor Emeritus of
Health Policy, University of California San Francisco, CA, USA

How Dr. Geyman does it is beyond me. He is one of the most prolific, scholarly, and courageous critics of US health care of our time. "The Future of US Health Care" is yet another of his invaluable contributions, full of illuminating facts, incisive analyses, and creative suggestions for a path forward. It belongs on the bookshelf of anyone who cares about the future of health care in America.

Donald M. Berwick, MD
President Emeritus and Senior Fellow
Institute for Healthcare Improvement, Boston, MA, USA

Contents

List of Tables ix

List of Figures xi

Preface xiii

PART 1: EVOLUTION OF U.S. HEALTH CARE SINCE THE 1960s 1

Chapter 1   Corporatization of Health Care Driving a Medical-Industrial Complex.............................3

Chapter 2   Evolution of the Private Health Insurance Industry 15

Chapter 3   New Medical Technologies: Impacts on the Costs of Health Care..................................25

Chapter 4   Increasing Privatization, Profiteering and Corruption..35

Chapter 5   Change of Values from a Service Ethic to a Business "Ethic" 45

PART 2: TODAY'S HEALTH CARE IN THE U.S. 55

Chapter 6   How Does U.S. Health Care Rank Internationally? 57

Chapter 7   Disparities, Inequities and Systemic Racism.................67

Chapter 8   Poor System Performance during the COVID Pandemic 77

Chapter 9   Failed Multi-Payer Financing Systems for U.S. Health Care 89

Chapter 10	How Wall Street and Corporate Interests Extract Profits and Professionalism from Health Care	99
Chapter 11	Barriers to System Reform	109

PART 3: MAJOR OPPOSING FUTURE SCENARIOS FOR REFORM OF HEALTH CARE 123

Chapter 12	"Free Market" Alternatives without Fundamental Reform	125
Chapter 13	Universal Coverage through National Health Insurance	135
Chapter 14	"Free Market" Profiteering vs. Not-for-Profit Patient Care: Which Will Prevail in 2040?	145

About the Author 161

Index 163

List of Tables

Table 1.1. Investor-owned care vs. not-for-profit care: Comparative examples 11
Table 2.1. Comparative features of privatized and public Medicare 19
Table 4.1. HMO "House calls": A new upcoding scam 39
Table 5.1. Fundamental principles of medical professionalism 47
Table 9.1. Why private health insurance is obsolete 95
Table 11.1. The vocabulary of health care 113
Table 12.1. Major problems of U.S. health care 126
Table 13.1. Alternative financing systems and American values 138
Table 13.2. Value-based comparison of four reform alternatives 140
Table 13.3. Evidence-based comparison of four reform alternatives 140
Table 14.1. Alternative scenarios for 2040 155

List of Figures

Figure 1.1.	Doctors spend twice as much time on EHR/desk work as with patients.	6
Figure 1.2.	Growth of physicians and administrators-1970-2019.	7
Figure 1.3.	Extent of for-profit ownership, 2016.	7
Figure 1.4.	Increasing burden of health care costs, 1980 – present.	8
Figure 1.5.	Milliman Medical Index, 2001-2019.	8
Figure 2.1.	Medicare overpays private plans.	20
Figure 2.2.	Medicare and Medicaid keep private insurers afloat.	20
Figure 2.3.	High deductibles cut all kinds of care.	21
Figure 3.1.	Influences on the use of new medical technology	26
Figure 3.2.	Pathways by which more medical care may lead to harm.	31
Figure 5.1.	Burnout strikes mid-career physicians hard.	50
Figure 6.1.	Overall ranking of eleven health care systems.	58
Figure 6.2.	Performance compared to health care spending.	59
Figure 6.3.	Cross national comparison of avoidable deaths.	59
Figure 6.4.	Insurance overhead, United States vs. five other countries, 2016.	61
Figure 6.5.	Rural hospital closures in America since 2010.	62
Figure 7.1.	The rise of the top 1% and fall of the bottom 50%, 1980-2016.	68
Figure 7.2.	Total United States population by race/ethnicity, 2019.	70
Figure 7.3.	Financial pain points during coronavirus outbreak: differ widely by race, ethnicity and income.	71
Figure 7.4.	Majority of Americans View our society as racist.	72
Figure 8.1.	Flattening the curve? No way in the USA	81
Figure 8.2.	Life expectancy fall from COVID-19: Greater in the U.S. than anyplace but Russia.	82
Figure 8.3.	State-by-state death toll from COVID, adjusted for population.	83

Figure 8.4. People of color in the U.S. were generally hit harder by the pandemic. 84
Figure 9.1. Workers' health insurance premiums are rising much faster than wages. 92
Figure 10.1. Total pe deals in healthcare: reported deal value, estimated deal value, and reported deal count, 2010-2020. ... 103
Figure 10.2. Private equity capital invested by segment: 2000-2019. 103
Figure 11.1. The great noise machine. 114
Figure 11.2. The Octopus Squeezing Congressional Debate and Action. 116
Figure 11.3. Too pig to fail. 117
Figure 11.4. The private-public revolving door as it perpetuates corporate interests. 118
Figure 12.1. Incremental reform doesn't fix U.S. health care. 131
Figure 13.1. Medicare for all savings compared to current system, 2019. 139
Figure 14.1. Federal campaign contributions from billionaires, 2000-2019. 150
Figure 14.2. Top 3 federal campaign contributors vs. all other billionaire contributors, 2000-2020. 151
Figure 14.3. Phoenix rising from the ashes. 157

Preface

For past generations, health care in the United States was a personal and community-based matter that didn't fill the news about unaffordable costs, barriers to care, and corporate profiteering. But those days are long gone as health care occupies the front burner of controversy and political debate. Now the most expensive health care system in the world, its high costs keep many millions of Americans from gaining access to care, which even then is variable and often poor quality. While we used to have a system more responsive to the public interest, today's dysfunctional system has been taken over by corporate stakeholders dedicated to their own profits rather than the care of patients and their families.

Although health care in the 1960s had its own problems, they were nothing like the degree of unaccountability that pervades U.S. health care today. Here are some markers of how today's health care is so different from the 1960s:

Then:

- Health care was a cottage industry without any corporate umbrella
- Most hospitals were community-based with local ownership
- Most physicians were self-employed with their own clinical autonomy
- Health care was a person and population-based service with a dominant service ethic

Now:

- Most health care is under corporatized ownership and management
- Most physicians and other health professionals are employed by others as "providers"
- We have seen a proliferation of investor-owned corporate chains

- Health care services have become a commodity for sale on an open market
- Profiteering, privatization, corruption and fraud are on the increase in health care markets

Having reached the nonagenarian age group with 60 years' experience in health care ranging from rural practice, teaching, administration and research, I feel both qualified and committed to writing this book. How this transformation has happened and accelerated over these six decades is an intriguing story from which we need to learn in order to improve and reform our system. Based on the above markers, we need to ask, and answer some fundamental questions that are still not yet being widely asked. The most basic question has become: Who is our health care system for—corporate stakeholders and Wall Street investors or the health and well-being of some 330 million Americans?

This book has three goals: (1) to bring historical perspective to how U.S. health care has evolved since the 1960s; (2) to describe and illustrate its many problems; and (3) to consider opportunities and obstacles to reform that will establish health care as an essential service for all Americans.

Part 1: Evolution of U.S. Health Care Since the 1960s

> *If we are to live comfortably with the new medical-industrial complex we must put our priorities together: the needs of patients and of society come first . . . How best to ensure that the medical-industrial complex serves the interests of patients first and of its shareholders second will have to be the responsibility of the medical profession and an informed public.*[1]
>
> —Arnold S. Relman, M.D., nephrologist, editor of *The New England Journal of Medicine* (1977 to 1991), and long-time advocate for physicians to retain an ethical commitment to patients and society.

---

[1] Relman, AS, e new medical-industrial complex. *N Engl J Med* 303: 969- 970, 1980.

Chapter 1

Corporatization of Health Care Driving a Medical-Industrial Complex

The last 60 years have seen a sea change in the way medicine is practiced in the United States and how our health care system has evolved. A corporate-based medical-industrial complex has risen over those years to be the dominant structure of our supposed "system" today. Here we have three goals: (1) to trace the development of the medical-industrial complex; (2) to describe how it has changed the culture of health care and medical practice; and (3) to consider the adverse impacts of this major change on patient care.

1. Rise of the Medical-Industrial Complex

Interestingly, concerns about the costs of medical care go way back to the Great Depression with a 1932 report by the Committee on the Costs of Medical Care (CCMC) making these recommendations that are still relevant today:

1. *Medical service should be furnished largely by organized groups.*
2. *Basic public health services should be extended so they will be available to the entire population according to its needs.*
3. *The costs of medical care should be placed on a group payment basis through the use of insurance or taxation or both* [1].

Blue Cross and Blue Shield were established in the 1930s on a non-profit and community rating basis (no exclusions for pre-existing conditions) whereby more people could afford care, with minimal out-of-pocket payments, and hospital beds could be kept open [2]. Following World War II and up to the mid-1960s, specialization of physicians was increasing, together with small private practices and independent hospitals at the center of U.S. health care.

Ironically, federal legislation enacting Medicare and Medicaid in 1965 played a large role in creating the medical-industrial complex that plagues health care today. New opportunities were opened up for corporate investment across the health care enterprise ranging from hospitals, nursing homes, clinical laboratories and the insurance industry. Hospitals were assured that their claims would be processed by Blue Cross as intermediaries [3]. From then on, the flood gates were open to ever increasing numbers of health care corporations and growing involvement of Wall Street interests. By 1984, the 8 largest investor-owned corporations together owned and operated 426 acute care hospitals, 102 psychiatric hospitals, 272 long-term care units, 62 dialysis centers, 89 ambulatory care centers, and a number of other ambulatory and home care services [4].

The first use of the term, *medical-industrial complex*, was in a 1970 book, *The American Health Empire: Power, Profits and Politics*, by John and Barbara Ehrenreich. They described the growth of technology and its products, replacement of physicians by hospitals at the center of a new system, and the increasing threat of institutionalized medicine to the doctor-patient relationship. They recommended that:

> *The health system should be re-created as a democratic enterprise, in which patients are participants (not customers or objects) and the health workers, from physicians to aides, are all colleagues in a common undertaking* [5].

The medical-industrial complex since then, however, has gained steam to become a corporate base for today's health care, including a shift to for-profit health care, privatization of public programs, and closer ties of corporations to investors. In his classic 1982 book, *The Social Transformation of American Medicine*, Paul Starr, Ph.D., Professor of Sociology at Princeton University observed:

> *The rise of a corporate ethos in medical care is already one of the most significant consequences of the changing structure of medical care. It permeates voluntary hospitals, government agencies, and academic thought as well as profit-making medical organizations . . . The organizational culture of medicine used to be dominated by the ideals of professionalism and voluntarism, which softened the underlying acquisitive activity. The restraint exercised by those ideals grew weaker. The "health center" of one era is the "profit center" of the next* [6].

Albert Jonsen, ethicist and author of *Clinical Ethics: A Practical Approach to Clinical Decisions in Clinical Medicine*, described the changed clinical environment in these terms:

> *The encounter between patient and physician is no longer a private place. It is a cubicle with open walls, surrounded by a crowd of managers, regulators, financiers, producers and lawyers required to manage the flow of money that makes that encounter possible. All of them can look into the encounter and see opportunities for profit or economy. All would like to have a say in how the encounter goes—from time consumed by it, to the drugs prescribed in it, to the costing out of each of its elements* [7].

2. Today's Culture of Medical Practice and Health Care

The marked differences in medical practice and health care between yesteryear and today can be encapsulated by these markers:

Then:

- Private practice was the norm;
- Physicians had their own paper charting system without computers;
- Physicians in private office practice also followed their patients in the hospital;
- Most practicing physicians had their own call system for after-hours care; and
- The prevailing ethic was one of service.

Now:

- Independent private practice is mostly gone, with more than two-thirds of physicians employed by others, mostly by hospital systems;
- Most hospital care is overseen by hospitalists who don't know their patients;
- Professionalism and clinical autonomy are threatened by pressure to be "productive" (i.e., bring in more revenue for your employer);
- Computerized electronic health records have become a billing instrument subject to profiteering by employers;

- Because of increased paper work, physicians have much less face-to-face time with their patients (Figure 1.1) [8].
- Increasing burnout, suicide and early retirements among physicians [9];
- Increasing barriers to care, with unaffordable costs and care based on ability to pay;
- Over-specialized physician workforce with primary care shortage;
- Marketing has replaced health care planning of earlier years;
- Public programs, such as Medicare and Medicaid, are increasingly privatized;
- Powerful forces are aligned to prevent regulation and reform; and
- The traditional ethic of service has been largely replaced by a business "ethic."

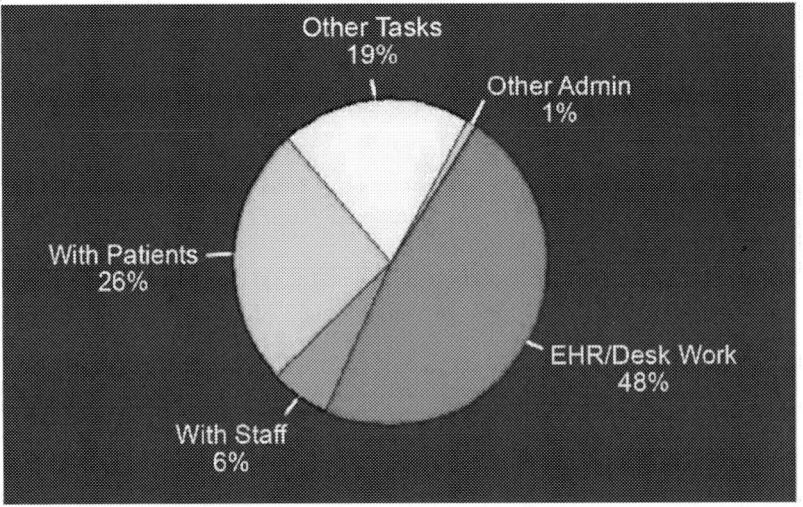

Source: Sinsky, C, Tutty, M, Colligan, L. Allocation of physician time in ambulatory practice. *Ann Intern Med* 166 (9): 683-684, 2017.

Figure 1.1. Doctors spend twice as much time on EHR/desk work as with patients.

A recent study of the time demands of the EHR are even more disturbing. U.S. physicians spend an average of 4.5 hours each practice day on it compared to just 1 hour in other countries. This high use lowers clinical focus, is inefficient, harms communication with patients and colleagues, and contributes to physician burnout [10].

As these trends have moved forward placing the pursuit of profits as the primary goal for corporatized health care, the numbers of administrators have grown exponentially compared to physicians, as shown in Figure 1.2 since 1970. Figure 1.3 shows the extent of for-profit ownership across the medical-industrial complex by 2016.

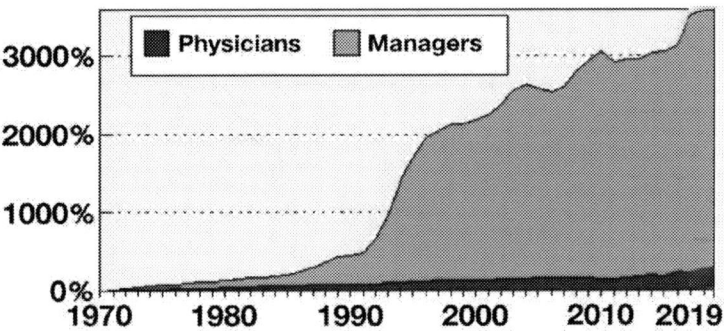

Source: Bureau of Labor Statistics; NCHS; and Himmelstein/Woolhandler analysis of CPS.
Note: Managers shown as moving average of current year and 2 previous years.

Figure 1.2. Growth of physicians and administrators-1970-2019.

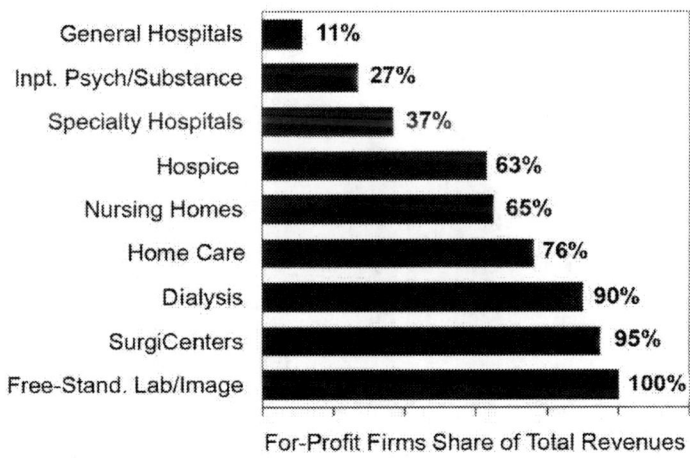

Source: Commerce Department, Service Annual Survey 2016 or most recent available data for share of establishments.

Figure 1.3. Extent of for-profit ownership, 2016.

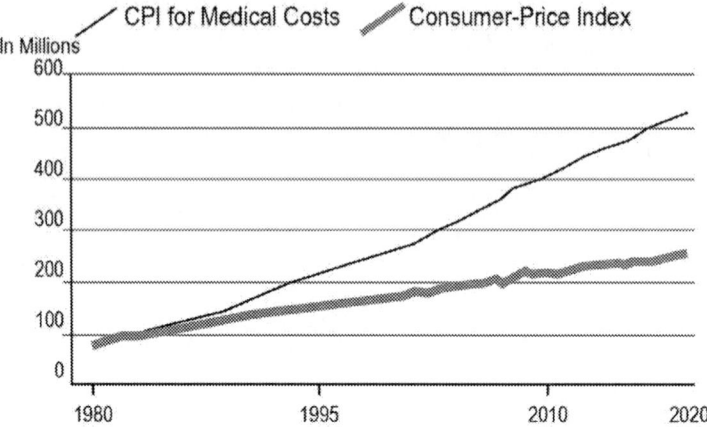

Source: Federal Reserve Bank of St. Louis.

Figure 1.4. Increasing burden of health care costs, 1980 – present.

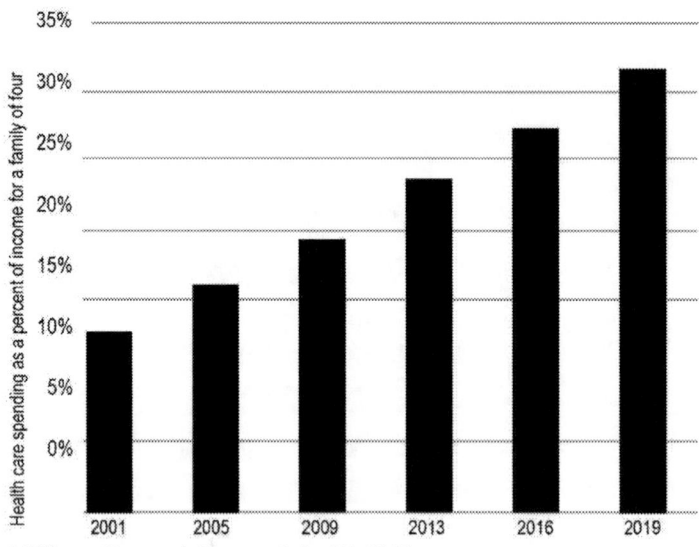

Source: Milliman Research Report, July 25, 2019.

Figure 1.5. Milliman Medical Index, 2001-2019.

The concern and need to contain health care prices that was recognized in the 1930s are still with us, never controlled in the public interest despite many legislative attempts to do so. Figure 1.4 shows the increasing burden of health care costs over the last 40 years, while Figure 1.5 shows how an average family of four, even when covered by an employer-sponsored preferred provider organization (PPO), now pays an average of more 30 percent of their annual income on health care [11].

The medical-industrial complex that now drives U.S. health care is a money-making machine that benefits corporate and Wall Street interests more than patients and the health professionals providing their care. The concerns raised by the Ehrenreichs in 1970 about uncontrollable health care costs plague us now and will into the future, while the basic questions asked in the Preface about the goals of our health care system remain unanswered.

There is a parallel between health care and the military-industrial complex, which President Dwight Eisenhower warned us about in his farewell address to the American people in 1961. Both complexes are beyond cost containment, with their goals unclear and increasing costs effectively lobbied to government payers. Andrew Cockburn, author of the 2021 book, *The Spoils of War; Power, Profit and the American War Machine*, tells us that the U.S. spends about $1 trillion a year on our war machine, without a clear objective. As he asks:

> *What is the objective? Is it to dominate the world and have 800 bases all around the world? Or is it to mount an effective defense against likely threats? In which case, we don't need very much. (His estimate in the latter case—maybe $100 billion a year). Commenting on the recent passage by Congress of a $778 billion defense bill with strong bipartisan support, he further observed that:*
>
> *On important matters, the electorate isn't you and me going to the polls. The real electorate are the major corporations, the major donors, the Wall Street banks* [12].

In health care, the electorate is an army of well-funded lobbyists promoting corporate interests across the medical-industrial complex, which are often at odds with the needs of the public.

3. Adverse Impacts of the Medical-Industrial Complex on Patient Care

The profit-driven medical-industrial complex, based on its goals and culture, continues to lead the way on the S & P 500 as it thwarts containment of prices and costs. As a result, patients, families, and taxpayers continue to incur these adverse impacts:

- prices to what the traffic will bear;
- decreased access to care due to unaffordable costs;
- variable, often poor quality of care;
- erosion of safety net sources of care; and
- rampant profiteering, even fraud.

Although market enthusiasts have for years assured us that an unfettered competitive marketplace can bring efficiency and cost containment in health care, that has been completely refuted by experience. The U.S. experiment with market-based medicine over the last four decades has enriched corporate stakeholders in the medical-industrial complex at the expense of patients, their families and taxpayers. Health care markets do not work in the same way as other markets for many reasons, such as patients often not knowing their needs, urgency of time, and non-transparency of costs. Perhaps most important, as predicted as early as 1963 by Kenneth Arrow, a leading economist at Columbia University, are the unavoidable uncertainties for both patients and physicians as to the diagnosis, treatment, and prognosis of illness [13].

Based on a nine-year study of 12 major health markets concluded in 2004, the non-partisan Center for Studying Health System Change found these four barriers preventing markets from being able to improve efficiency and quality of care: (1) providers' market power; (2) absence of potentially efficient provider systems; (3) employers' inability to push the system toward efficiency and quality; and (4) insufficient health plan competition [14]. If the above is not enough to bury the myth that effective competition exists in an unfettered health care marketplace, the experience with investor-owned health care corporations across the medical-industrial complex does so without any question. As Table 1.1 shows, their track record has been undeniably poor regardless of the part of the health care system involved [15-25].

Table 1.1. Investor-owned care vs. not-for-profit care: Comparative examples

Hospitals	Higher costs, fewer nurses, and higher death rates [15,16]
Emergency medical services	Higher prices, worse care with slower response times. [17]
HMOs	Worse scores on all 14 quality of care measures. [18]
Nursing homes	Often in corporate chains, have lower staffing levels, worse quality of care, and higher death rates. [19]
Mental health centers	Restrictive barriers and limits to care, such as premature discharge without adequate outpatient care. [20]
Dialysis centers	Mortality rates 19 to 24 percent higher;[21] 53 percent less likely to be put on a transplant waiting list. [22]
Assisted living facilities	Many critical incidents of physical, emotional, or sexual abuse of patients. [23]
Home health agencies	Higher costs, lower quality of care. [24]
Hospice	Missed visits and neglect of patients dying at home. [25]

Source: Geyman, JP. *The Corrosion of Medicine: Can the Profession Reclaim Its Moral Legacy?* Monroe, ME. *Common Courage Press,* 2008, p. 37.

Conclusion

The foregoing makes a compelling case that the U.S. health care system is held captive by corporate stakeholders in our medical-industrial complex to the detriment of the health of our population. With by far the most expensive health care in the world, essential care is beyond the reach of 30 million uninsured and 87 million underinsured Americans. If and when they can get care, their outcomes are worse than their counterparts in many other countries around the world. Moreover, as taxpayers, we are far from getting our money's worth in health care.

We have seen an ongoing political battle between corporate interests, their investors and allies over how health care should be provided and the role of government in ensuring that we have a system that meets the needs of all Americans. No end is yet in sight as to whether and when significant reform can be achieved in the public interest. Later chapters will delve into system problems and what can be done about them. But for now we turn to the next chapter where we will see whether and if the private insurance industry protects us from the unavoidable health risks that we all have.

References

[1] Falk, IS. Some lessons from the fifty years since the COMC Final Report, 1932. *J Public Health Policy* 4 (2): 139, 1983.
[2] McNerny, W. C Rufus Rorem award lecture. Big question for the Blues: Where to go from here? *Inquiry.* (Summer): 33: 110-117, 1996.
[3] Andrews, C. *Profit fever: The Drive to Corporatize Health Care and How to Stop It.* Monroe, ME. *Common Courage Press*, 1995.
[4] Gray, BE (Ed.) *For-Profit Enterprise in Health Care: Supplementary Statement on For-Profit Enterprise in Health Care.* Washington, D.C. *National Academy Press*, 1986.
[5] Ehrenreich, B and J. The Medical-Industrial Complex. Review of book by Ginzberg, E (with Ostow, M) *Men, Money and Medicine. The New York Review of Books.* New York, Columbia, 1970.
[6] Starr, P. *The Social Transformation of American Medicine.* New York. *Basic Books*, 1982, p. 448.
[7] Jonsen, A. Opening remarks, Symposium on Commercialism in Medicine, Program in Medicine & Human Values. California Pacific Medical Center, San Francisco: September 2005. *Cambridge Quarterly of Health Care*, spring 2007.
[8] Sinsky, C, Tutty, M, Colligan, L. Allocation of physician time in ambulatory practice. *Ann Intern Med* 166 (9): 683-684, 2017.
[9] Abbott, B. Burnout strikes mid-career physicians hard. *Wall Street Journal*, January 16, 2020: A 3.
[10] Gogineni, T, Kahn, JG, Maya, S. How much time do physicians spend in the EHR? *KevinMD.com*, April 10, 2022.
[11] Girod, CS, Hart, SK, Liner, DM. 2019 Milliman Medical Index. *Milliman Research Report*, December 2019.
[12] Cockburn, A. Power, profit and the American war machine. As interviewed by *Corporate Crime Reporter* 36 (3), January 17, 2022.
[13] Arrow, KJ. Uncertainty and the welfare economics of medical care. *American Economic Review* 53: 941-973, 1963.

[14] Nichols, LM, Ginsburg, PB, Berenson, RA, Christianson, J, & Hurley, RE. Are market forces strong enough to deliver efficient health care systems? Confidence is waning. *Health Aff (Millwood)* 23 (2): 8-11, 2004.
[15] Silverman, EM, Skinner, JS, & Fisher, ES. The association between for-profit hospital ownership and increased Medicare spending. *N Engl J Med* 341: 420, 1999.
[16] Woolhandler, S, Himmelstein, DU. Costs of care and administration at for-profit and other hospitals in the United States. *N Engl J Med* 36: 769, 1997.
[17] Ivory, D, Protess, B, Daniel, J. When you dial 911 and Wall Street answers. *New York Times*, June 25, 2016.
[18] Himmelstein, DU, S Woolhandler, I Hellander, S M Wolfe. Quality of care in investor-owned vs not-for-profit HMOs. *JAMA* 282: 159, 1999.
[19] Harrington, C, Steffie Woolhandler, Joseph Mullan, Helen Carrillo and David U. Himmelstein. Does investor-ownership of nursing homes compromise the quality of care? *Am J Public Health* 91 (9): 1, 2001.
[20] Munoz, R. How health care insurers avoid treating mental illness. *San Diego Union Tribune*, May 22, 2002.
[21] Devereaux, PJ, Schünemann, HJ, Ravindran, N, Bhandari, M, Garg, AX, Choi, PT-L, Grant, BJB, Haines, T, Lacchetti, C, Weaver, B, Lavis, JN, Cook, DJ, Haslam, DRS, Sullivan, T, & Guyatt, GH. Comparison of mortality between for-profit and private not-for-profit hemodialysis centers: A systematic review and meta-analysis. *JAMA* 288: 2449, 2002.
[22] Garg, PP, Frick, KD, Diener-West, M, & Powe, NR. Effect of the ownership of dialysis facilities on patients' survival and referral for transplantation. *N Engl J Med* 341: 1653, 1999.
[23] Pear, R. U.S. pays billions for 'assisted living,' but what does it get? *New York Times*, February 18, 2018.
[24] Cabin, W, Himmelstein, DU, Siman, ML, Woolhandler, S. For profit Medicare home health agencies' costs appear higher and quality appears lower compared to not-for-profit agencies. *Health Affairs* 33 (8): 1460-1465, 2014.
[25] Waldman, P. Preparing Americans for death lets hospices neglect end of life. *Bloomberg*, July 22, 2011.

Chapter 2

Evolution of the Private Health Insurance Industry

> *The United States subscribes to a business model that characterizes insurers as commercial entities. Like all businesses, their goal is to make money... Under the business model, casual inhumanity is built in and the common good ignored. Excluding the poor, the aged, the disabled, and the ill is sound policy since it maximizes profit. Under the social model, denying coverage to any member of society would refute the fundamental purpose of health insurance* [1].
>
> —Bernard Lown, M.D., Cardiologist, developer of the cardiac defibrillator, Professor Emeritus at the Harvard School of Public Health, author of *The Lost Art of Healing: Practicing Compassion in Medicine*, and co-recipient of the Nobel Peace Prize in 1985 on behalf of International Physicians for the Prevention of Nuclear War, which he co-founded.

That quote by the distinguished Dr. Lown highlights a core issue for insuring health care in this country, which is still unresolved. In their earlier years, private insurers served their clients well, but that was to change after the 1960s as our experiment with an unfettered health care marketplace took hold within the medical-industrial complex. The goals of this chapter are (1) to bring historical perspective to the origins of private health insurance in the U.S. from its not-for-profit origins to its profiteering role today; (2) to describe its stages of development to the point of its current failure to provide protection for its enrollees at affordable costs; and (3) to consider potential options whereby the financing base of our health care system can be stabilized.

1. Historical Perspective

This statement sets the stage for the urgent need for health insurance. Can you guess when it was made?

> *The high cost of health care has created a real burden for the great financial middle class, composed of self-respecting people who are too proud to accept free service and too poor to be able to afford the costly private rooms, highly paid surgeons and the expensive laboratory studies that have done so much to take guesswork out of modern medicine and surgery* [2].

If you said some time in the last 40 or 50 years, you would have missed it. It was in 1926 in an issue of the *Saturday Evening Post*! That's how long the challenge of affording health care in this country has existed.

Not long after that, help was on the way during the Great Depression in Dallas, Texas, where Baylor University's University Hospital was deeply in debt with over one-third of its general hospital beds empty. A prepaid group hospital plan was developed for more than 1,300 Dallas teachers, which became a prototype for later Blue Cross plans. It provided free hospitalization for up to 21 days a year as well as coverage for operating room, laboratory and anesthesia services, whereby the Hospital was paid directly without a third party [3]. By 1935, major multi-hospital Blue Cross plans were operational in Durham, North Carolina, Washington, D.C., and Cleveland, Ohio; the Durham plan was the first to provide complete dependent coverage [4]. By 1940, with the goal to share risk across a broad risk pool, there were 39 state-based Blue Cross plans with an enrollment of more than 6 million people [5].

World War II then became the main impetus for the rapid development of employer-sponsored health insurance (ESI). A wartime economy had brought the country out of the Depression and into a severe labor shortage, so that employers had to compete for workers by offering higher pay and/or fringe benefits. IRS rulings helped by allowing employers tax exemptions for the costs of health insurance while letting those benefits be non-taxable for employees [6].

The health insurance market became intensely competitive after World War II as large numbers of for-profit commercial insurers entered an expanding workplace ESI market. Darwinian competition developed whereby commercial insurers attracted many enrollees away from the not-for-profit Blues by reducing premiums for lower-risk enrollees and by offering limited indemnity coverage that avoided the high costs of hospital care. The number of insured Americans grew from 77 million in 1950 to 132 million in 1960 as commercial insurers gained the largest share of that surge [7].

2. Growth of Private Health Insurance: Leaving Its Roots for Maximal Profits

2.1. Shift from Not-for-Profit to for-Profit

In the face of fierce competition, the Blues were under pressure to compromise their earlier service mission and experiment with experience rating and indemnity coverage, especially in the individual non-group market. In their earlier not-for-profit plans, *community rating* had been the norm, whereby risk was shared across all enrollees in the covered population at the same premium. *Guaranteed issue* had also been part of their plans, with coverage being offered to all comers.

Experience rating and medical underwriting became the new way for the Blues to compete against commercial insurers, who had become expert at separating out healthier enrollees from higher risk individuals and groups for coverage. There were many ways to do that, including setting age limits and denial of coverage based on pre-existing conditions. Thomas Kinser, chief operating officer of the Blue Cross Blue Shield Association, described the process this way in 1992:

> *With modern electronic data processing technology and new rating methods, these cherry-picking companies can—under the current rules [and] with full blessing of insurance commissions—find good risks, raise rates enormously if they get claims at the end of the first year, and have a pool of business that they [profit from] . . . But they are not looking for stability of relationships with customers, predictable financing, and good community health systems* [8].

By 2005, one-half of the nation's Blue Cross Blue Shield plans had been consolidated and converted into for-profit companies [9]. As intense competition among insurers was off and running, the following techniques became ways to extract more income at the expense of reliable and affordable coverage for enrollees. Note how in each instance the industry gets larger and more powerful in market share and politically with closer ties to Wall Street investors.

2.1.1. Growth of a Denial Industry

In order to increase their profits, private insurers try to initially deny coverage of higher-risk people. They have many ways to do this, including holding marketing meetings on the second floor of buildings without elevators to discourage less mobile and older people. When confronted by claims from enrollees sicker than expected, they just make steep increases in their premiums, such as by 62 percent in Tennessee [10] and 116 percent in Arizona in 2016 [11]. Once covered, denial of claims through burdensome preauthorization of services is activated as another way to avoid paying expensive claims. That process has further increased the bureaucracy, to the point that U.S. nurses have been spending more than 13 hours a week to obtain prior authorizations, compared to none in Canada with its single-payer system [12]. Today, the average denial rate for in-network claims submitted by providers under the Affordable Care Act is 18 percent [13].

2.1.2. Managed Care

As a new effort to contain health care costs, managed care grew rapidly during and after the 1990s. It changed payment for health care services from fee-for-service to prospective payment based on capitation, the number of individual enrollees in a health plan, regardless of the amount of care provided. It was really more about managed *reimbursement* than care, easily manipulated by insurers owning health maintenance organizations (HMOs) for higher profits. Cutting down on prospective payments increased physicians' workload, more denial of services, and worse care. By 2000, 65 million Americans were enrolled in HMOs, and almost 80 percent of physicians had at least one managed care contract [14].

2.1.3. Privatization of Public Programs

Both Medicare and Medicaid have been increasingly privatized in recent years as insurers seek to exploit solid federal funding sources. Compared with traditional public Medicare, privatized Medicare costs more, is more inefficient, more restrictive of choice, more volatile (plans can leave a market with little notice), and have an administrative overhead five or six times higher than for traditional Medicare. Table 2.1 shows the basic differences between privatized Medicare and traditional public Medicare as of the early 2000s [15].

Table 2.1. Comparative features of privatized and public Medicare

PRIVATIZED MEDICARE	ORIGINAL MEDICARE
Experience-rated eligibility	Universal coverage
Managed competition	Social insurance as earned right
Defined contribution	Defined benefits
Segmented risk pool	Broad risk pool
Market pricing to risk	Administered prices
More volatile access & benefits	More reliable access & benefits
Increased cost sharing	Less cost sharing
Less accountability	Potential for more accountability
Less choice of provider & hospital	Full choice of provider & hospital
Less well distributed	Well distributed
Less efficiency, higher overhead	More efficiency, lower overhead

Source: Geyman, JP., "Shredding the Social Contract: The Privatization of Medicare." Monroe, ME. *Common Courage Press,* 2006, p.206.

One typical way used by insurers to increase their revenues is by up-coding diagnoses, thereby exaggerating how sick their enrollees are and claiming payment for conditions for which care was not provided [16]. As a result of these kinds of practices, the federal government has been overpaying insurers for many years, even with increases since the Affordable Care Act (ACA) was passed in 2020 (Figure 2.1) [17]. Overpayments to private Medicaid managed care plans are endemic in more than 30 states, frequently involving unnecessary and duplicative payments to providers [18].

Recent years have seen increasingly egregious exploitation of seniors through investor-owned direct contracting entities as middlemen for Medicare Advantage. A little-known federal agency, the Center for Medicare and Medicaid Innovation, has been moving enrollees, without their consent, to supposed "risk bearing" for-profit middlemen known as Direct Contracting Entities (DCEs). The goal: to gain further profits from Medicare (already more than 40 percent privatized) through increased overpayments to private insurers, threatening the future Medicare funding while allowing the insurance industry to pose as risk-bearing while taxpayers are really the ones at risk [19]. As Figure 2.2 shows, profits from privatized Medicare and Medicaid have been the lifeblood of private insurers [20].

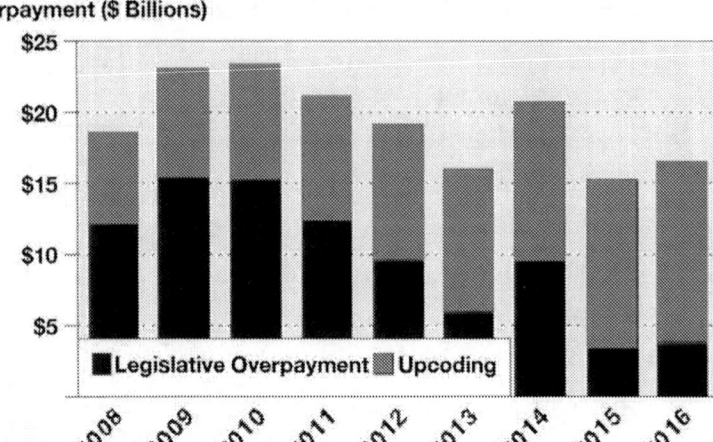

Source: PNHP Report 10/20/12 - based on data from MedPAC, *Comonwealth Fund*, Trivedi et al.

Figure 2.1. Medicare overpays private plans.

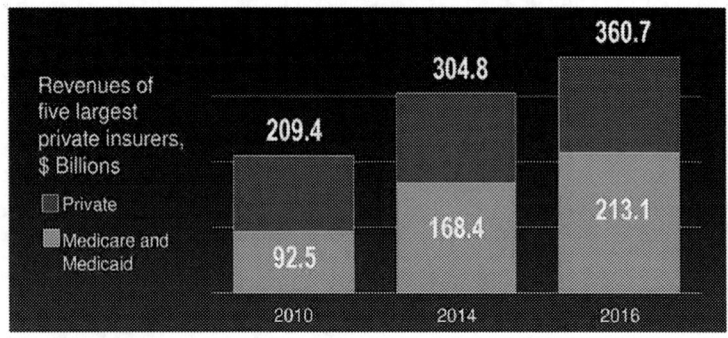

Source: *Health Affairs;* 36 (2):185, 2017.

Figure 2.2. Medicare and Medicaid keep private insurers afloat.

2.1.4. Consolidation with Growing Market Power

Mergers and consolidation within the private health insurance industry have been proceeding apace since the 1990s, and actually accelerated after passage of the ACA. In each instance, this means higher market shares, less competition, higher costs, less options, and less protection for enrollees. A 2021 report found that health insurer consolidation had grown by 56 percent from 2014 and 2020. The largest health insurers (in numeric order—United

Health Group, Anthem, Aetna and Cigna) together had a market share of 48 percent, while the Blues in 2018 dominated ACA exchanges with a market share of almost 50 percent [21]. This level of consolidation brings with it more cost-sharing with higher deductibles, reduced access and utilization of care across the board (Figure 2.3) [22].

Profits to insurers can reach astounding levels, even without growth of enrolled numbers of patients. As one example, United Health reported profits of $24 billion in 2021, with most of its revenue from the company's Medicare Advantage plans and state Medicaid programs that it manages and no growth in the numbers of enrollees [23].

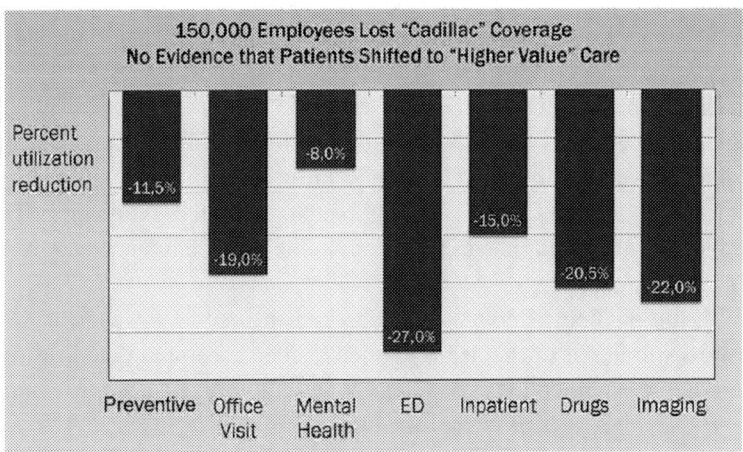

Source: Brot-Goldberg et al. June, 2015.

Figure 2.3. High deductibles cut all kinds of care.

2.1.5. Growing Reach of Health Insurers into Other Parts of the Medical-Industrial Complex

In recent years, giant insurers have been extending their reach across the medical-industrial complex by purchasing companies in health information technology, physician management, and other areas that give them more clout and market share in their favor. United Health Group, the largest insurer by revenue, sells technology to hospitals, manages clinical trials, distributes prescription drugs, and offers continuing medical education to physicians [24]. Recently, through its Optum health services arm, it has acquired LHC Group Inc, one of the largest home health firms in the country, adding to its portfolio that already includes physician groups, clinics and surgery centers [25].

3. Potential Approaches to Stabilize Health Care Financing

The private multi-payer health insurance industry in this country sold out to Wall Street investors years ago as it has gamed the system in many ways, ranging from deceptive marketing and denial of services to ever higher cost sharing, restricted networks, and limited drug formularies. Most people are unaware of the extent of federal funding along the way, including an average annual subsidy of $685 billion [26] and overpayments as shown in Figure 2.1 [27]. The private health insurance industry does all this by providing worse access, increased denials of services, worse quality of care, less reliability by exiting less profitable markets—all with excessive administrative overhead.

The COVID-19 pandemic has wrought major changes in the U.S. workplace that place the future of employer sponsored insurance (ESI) in doubt. Before the pandemic, ESI had the single largest share of private health insurance in the country, insuring about 150 million Americans. During the pandemic, however, job losses left many millions uninsured with many jobs lost indefinitely. Other factors pointing to changes further reducing ESI in the future include more people working from home and the replacement of many jobs by robots.

With the decline of employer-sponsored insurance, the industry is in a downward spiral. All of that leads Wendel Potter, a former Vice President of Corporate Communications at CIGNA and author of *Deadly Spin: An Insurance Company Insider Speaks Out on How Corporate PR Is Killing Health Care and Deceiving Americans*, to this well-grounded conclusion in 2019:

> *Our health insurance companies are not essential. They don't treat anyone. They don't prevent anyone from becoming sick. They don't take you to the hospital or make sure you take your pills. They don't discover medical innovations. They're simply middlemen we don't need. And in the industry, we always dreaded the day American businesses and patients would wake up to that reality. That day has come* [28].

Now that the COVID pandemic has revealed the inadequacy of ESI as a foundation of U.S. health insurance, it is time to explore alternatives that are affordable to patients, families and taxpayers. As we will discuss in Chapter 13, we have four major alternatives before us: (1) building on the ACA; (2) some kind of a public option; (3) Medicare Advantage for All; and (4) improved Medicare for All (the only option that would provide universal coverage and has a high level of popular support) [29].

Conclusion

We will further consider the failure of our multi-payer financing system of U.S. health care in Chapter 9. Until then, we turn next to the story of how technology advances have led to escalation of health care costs as well as becoming commodities on a growing market for investors on the backs of patients.

References

[1] Lown, B. Physicians need to fight the business model of medicine. *Hippocrates* 12 (5): 25-28, 1998.
[2] Editorial on health care costs in a 1926 issue of *Saturday Evening Post* as cited in: *Proceedings of Spring Meeting of Society of Actuaries,* Spring 2007.
[3] Stuart, JE. *The Blue Cross Story: An Informal Biography of the Voluntary Nonprofit Prepayment Plan for Hospital Care.* Chicago: BCBSA Archives.
[4] Ibid # 3, pp 29-30.
[5] Somers, HM & Somers, AR. *Doctors, Patients and Health Insurance.* Washington, D.C.: The Brookings Institution, 1961, p, 548.
[6] Ibid # 5, pp. 109-111.
[7] Andrews, C. *Profit Fever: The Drive to Corporatize Health Care and How to Stop It.* Monroe, ME. *Common Courage Press*, 1995, pp. 3-8.
[8] Cunningham, RC III, Cunningham, RM, Jr. *The Blues: A History of the Blue Cross and Blue Shield System.* DeKalb, IL. *The Northern Illinois University Press*, 1997, pp. 35-36.
[9] Schramm, C. The diseconomies of Blue Cross conversion. Washington, D.C.: *Alliance for Advancing Non-Profit Health Care.*, February, 2005.
[10] Radnofsky, L, Armour, S. States approve steep health-premium increases. *Wall Street Journal*, August 24, 2016.
[11] Montgomery, D. Minnesota's health insurance premium hike is fourth-highest in nation. *Pioneer Press*, October 24, 2016.
[12] Morra, D, Nicholson, S, Levinson, W, Gans, DN, Hammons, T, Casalino, LP. U.S. physician practices versus Canadians: spending nearly four times as much money interacting with payers. *Health Affairs* 30 (8): 1443-1450, 2011.
[13] Silvers, JB. This is the most realistic path to Medicare for All. *New York Times*, October 16, 2019.

[14] Jensen, G A, Michael A Morrisey, Shannon Gaffney, and Derek K Liston. The new dominance of managed care: Insurance trends in the 1990s. *Health Affairs (Millwood)* 16 (1): 125-136, 1997.
[15] Geyman, JP. *Shredding the Social Contract: The Privatization of Medicare*. Monroe, ME. *Common Courage Press*, 2006, p. 206.
[16] Livingston, S. Insurers profit from Medicare Advantage's incentive to add coding that boosts reimbursement. *Modern Healthcare*, September 4, 2018.
[17] Geruso, M, Layton, T. Up-coding inflates Medicare costs in excess of $2 billion annually. *UT News*, University of Texas at Austin, June 18, 2015.
[18] Herman, B. Medicaid's unmanaged managed care. *Modern Healthcare*, April 30, 2016.
[19] Malinow, A. An obscure agency is threatening to hand Medicare over to Wall Street. *Truthout*, December 3, 2021.
[20] Schoen, C, Collins, SR. The Big Five health insurers' membership and revenue trends: Implications for public policy. *Health Affairs* 36 (2), December, 2017.
[21] Waddill, K. Health insurance consolidation grew from 2014 to 2020. *Health Payer Intelligence*, September 29, 2021.
[22] Shankaran, V. as quoted by Stallings, E. High-deductible health policies linked to delayed diagnosis and treatment. *NPR*, April 18, 2019.
[23] While United Health reports $24 billion in profits, Americans faced 200% increases in out-of-pocket costs over last decade. *Wendell Potter NOW*, January 21 2022.
[24] Murphy, T. United Health looks beyond insurance to help fuel 4Q growth. *Associated Press*, January 17, 2017.
[25] Mathews, AW. United Health to buy home health firm LHC Group for $5.4 billion. *Wall Street Journal*, March 29, 2022.
[26] Ockerman, E. It costs $685 billion a year to subsidize U.S. health insurance. *Bloomberg News*, May 23, 2018.
[27] Ibid # 17.
[28] Potter, W. Why the private health insurance industry faces an existential crisis. *The Progressive Populist*, November 1, 2019, p. 9.
[29] Geyman, JP. The future of work in America: Demise of employer-sponsored insurance and what should replace it. *Intl J Health Services*, October 20, 2021.

Chapter 3

New Medical Technologies: Impacts on the Costs of Health Care

Be careful about reading health books; you may die of a misprint.
—Mark Twain

Mark Twain's concern about the risk of reading health books translates to today's times when reading about new medical technologies. The deeper that you get into this subject, the more you find yourself enveloped by controversies over risks vs. possible benefits for individuals vs. populations, as well as potential costs to individuals, families, taxpayers, and society. In the first chapter, we saw some of the many ways that the U.S. leads the way in high prices and costs of health care, still largely uncontained in a Wall Street based medical-industrial complex. In the second chapter, we saw how our mostly for-profit health insurance industry thrives by avoiding protection of higher-risk individuals.

We already know that new technologies often have a way of generating higher costs to go with their high expectations, so how can we deal with potential further uncontrolled increases in costs and prices that are already unaffordable? This chapter will try to answer that question with five goals: (1) to consider the influences that relate to advancing new technologies; (2) to show how these technologies inflate prices and costs of health care; (3) to describe how new technologies are evaluated and approved; (4) to consider whether they are worth it; and (5) to briefly discuss lessons from here and abroad about controlling the costs of new technologies while improving the health of all Americans.

1. Pressures to Bring New Technologies to U.S. Health Care

In their classic book, *Hope or Hype: The Obsession with Medical Advances and the High Cost of False Promises*, Drs. Richard Deyo and

Donald Patrick, former colleagues at the University of Washington, bring us these myths about new technologies:

- "Newer is always better;
- "Experimental" and "standard" care are well defined;
- Doctors adopt medical advances only on the basis of good science;
- More medical tests are always better; information can only be good;
- Action is always better than inaction;
- Doctors adopt new treatments only if those treatments offer good value for money;
- We can cure most medical conditions [1]."

These myths are pervasive and have much to do with the diverse kinds of medical "advances" that are brought forward, some of which are useful but many of which turn out to be detrimental, some even harmful. How to sort them out is a challenge. There is always strong pressure from within a corporatized medical establishment to favor more than less. Figure 3.1 shows how many influences are involved in considering what technologies are actually brought to market and use [2].

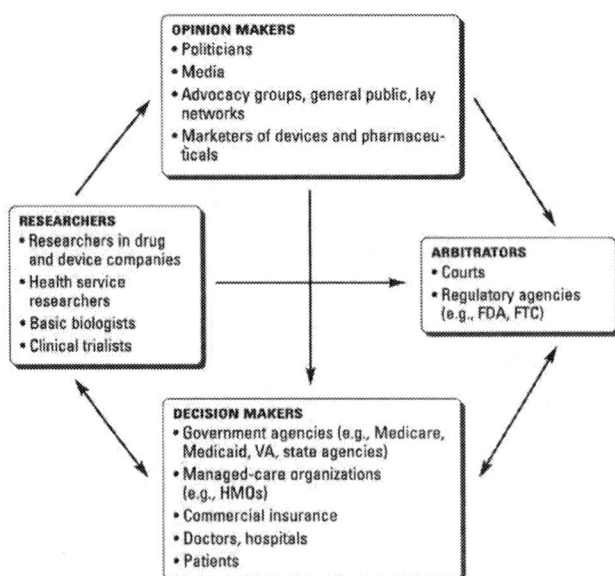

Source: Reproduced with permission from R. A. Deyo, *Annual Review of Public Health*, 2002.

Figure 3.1. Influences on the use of new medical technology.

Whereas we might assume that advances in science are the main drivers of new technologies, that is often not true. Corporate interests, their lobbyists, and some in government can promote some "advances" on the basis of their market value without solid scientific evidence of their value to patients and populations. They can also oppose and defeat efforts by government to evaluate the value of potential advances. The U.S. has a long line of starts and stops of federal agencies that succumbed to this pressure, including the National Center for Health Care Technology (1978-1981) and the Office of Technology Assessment (1972-1995).

2. How New Technologies Inflate Health Care Costs

These are just some of many drivers of higher prices and costs of new medical technologies, many of which are below the radar of public awareness:

- Corporate interests building momentum for future markets for their products through media hype of marketing studies disguised as "research."
- Collusion of some physicians with industry who take large amounts of money for promotional talks and "consulting" that are really disguised marketing strategies. As one example, a 2019 report found that at least 500 U.S. physicians had taken in at least $500,000 in the last five years from drug and medical device companies for this purpose, with more than 700 receiving more than $1 million each [3].
- Secret deals between drug manufacturers and pharmacy benefit managers, such as CVS Caremark and Express Scripts, that drive up prices for prescription drugs as they accelerate through corporate mergers [4].
- Direct to consumer drug advertising, adopted in this country in 1993 but not permitted in other advanced countries because of bias rather than science.
- Commodification of screening, testing, and procedures as billable services further drives up health care costs.
- Wearable devices (e.g., the new Apple Watch), without established cost-benefit that check on heart rhythms to detect atrial fibrillation, but will inflate costs to reach a clinical diagnosis [5].

- Once established, the cost of drugs, as with other services, can increase markedly without explanation except for profiteering. There are many such examples, including the exorbitant increase of Daraprim used by patients with HIV from $13.50 to $750 per tablet in 2017 [6], to steep cost increases by Eli Lilly & Co. of its popular Humalog injections that force many diabetics to pay up to $1,200 for a life-saving drug [7]. A 2019 report found that the U.S. paid more than $5 billion during 2017 and 2018 for wild price increases of drugs without evidence of benefit to patients [8].

3. Evaluation and Approval Process for New Technologies

A major contributor to the high costs of new technologies in the U.S. is the fact that costs are not dealt with directly in the evaluation and approval process. As Deyo and Patrick observed 15 years ago:

> *We generally avoid deciding what's too expensive, and agree to cover nearly everything that offers even trivial benefits. This prices more and more people out of any health insurance and increases the amount you have to pay out of pocket. If health care costs keep rising much faster than inflation, the logical extension is that at some point our entire national wealth will go for health care. At some point, we may collectively decide that this isn't the best strategy* [9].

That observation is still spot on as we have made no progress in dealing with this challenge. The recent accelerated approval by the FDA of Aduhelm (aducanumab), a new drug for the treatment of Alzheimer's dementia, is yet another example that we still pay no attention to cost. Against the advice of an advisory committee, the FDA went with another of its committees to grant *accelerated* approval based on the likelihood (not yet demonstrated) that it will have clinical benefits to patients. At that point, Biogen, its manufacturer, set its *wholesale* price at $56,000 a year, which it was forced to reduce to $28,000 after receiving widespread bad press for such a price. The accelerated approval process also received intense criticism for lacking evidence of Aduhelm's efficacy and potential risks. The FDA is still requiring Biogen to conduct a post-approval clinical trial to verify the drug's clinical benefit, and could take steps to remove it from the market if it is not sufficiently effective [10].

Meanwhile, Medicare has recently decided to deny routine payment for the drug unless patients are enrolled in clinical trials for the drug [11].

In contrast to other advanced countries, the U.S. does not use cost-effectiveness analysis, a well-developed technique, as part of the evaluation and approval of new treatments, largely due to continued opposition from industry. Moreover, the drug and medical device industries have long resisted price controls and opposed regulation of the safety of their products, as these examples illustrate:

- *The drug industry:* It has coopted effective regulation by paying more than $2 billion a year in user fees to the FDA, for which it gets industry-friendly policies that include accelerated drug approvals without proven evidence of a new drug's efficacy and safety. Many reviewers on FDA panels have close ties to industry and one-half of health care lobbyists are former government officials [12]. A 2016 report found that unsafe FDA-approved drugs were prescribed more than 100 million times between 1993 and 2010 before they were recalled from the market [13].
- *The medical device industry* also has a friendly relationship with the FDA, which requires only "substantial equivalence" to other similar devices instead of evidence of effectiveness and safety. Not surprisingly, a 2003 study found that more than 1,000 medical devices were being recalled each year as a threat to public safety [14]. Johnson & Johnson's all-metal hip prosthesis was finally withdrawn from the market after failure rates in the U.S. and abroad led to some 5,000 lawsuits against the company, but it still continued to be sold overseas [15].

4. Are These New Technologies Worth It?

From the above, we can realize that many new technologies are *not* worth it. We can also see the complexity of the process by which new technologies are evaluated. Further complexity is added by what will happen to their prices and costs into the future, which bears directly upon their affordability by patients/families and government.

Lewis Thomas, well-known physician, researcher, writer and administrator (including Dean of Yale Medical School), described three levels of medical technology that help to clarify the terrain of our question:

- *non-technology*: palliative care for patients with advanced diseases, such as cancer, without hope of cure or changing the course of the disease.
- *halfway technology*: noncurative but able to improve quality of life or delay death, such as kidney dialysis.
- *high technology*: curative treatments or effective preventive services, such as the polio and smallpox vaccines [16].

By that classification, we have to admit that many of the medical technologies in use today are halfway technologies without the potential for cures. In terms of affordability, there are also many examples of technologies that have become unaffordable through profiteering at the point of care. What has happened with electronic medical records comes to mind—beyond its original purpose of providing essential information to health care professionals about patients, it has become a billing instrument as a revenue-building tool for providers (most often hospital systems), thereby increasing costs to payers and patients.

New technologies are often a double-edged sword, as shown by the introduction of CT scanning. True, it has been a useful advance, but is frequently overused by hospitals, adding unaffordable costs to patients' bills, and leading to further testing and costs to patients in pursuit of incidental findings that are often clinically insignificant. As just two examples of the extent of this problem, a 2016 report found that 40 to 70 percent of CT scans of the abdomen and 40 percent of CT scans of the lumbar spine found such incidental findings [17].

At the macro system level, Drs. Elliott Fisher and Gilbert Welch at Dartmouth Medical School's Center for the Evaluative Clinical Sciences, have called attention to the many ways that more medical care can lead to harm, including financial impacts on payers and patients. (Figure 3.2) [18] Beyond the growth of new technologies, there are two other important drivers of transformational change that inflate the cost of medical care—medicalization of preventive and therapeutic services and promotion leading to increased demand for services, whether necessary or not.

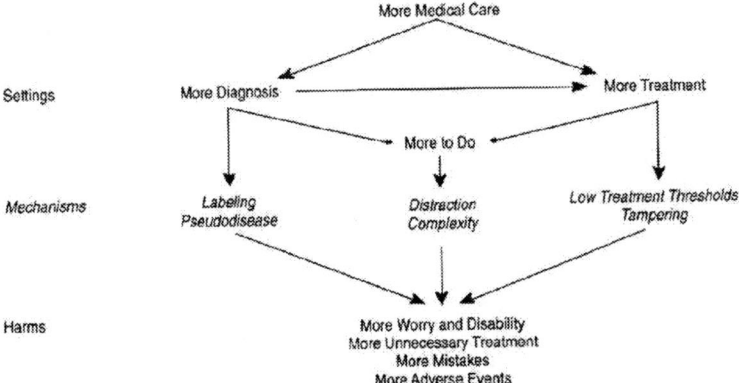

Source: Fisher, ES, Welch, HG. Avoiding the unintended consequences of growth in medical care: How might more be worse? *JAMA* 281:446-453, 1999.

Figure 3.2. Pathways by which more medical care may lead to harm.

5. What Lessons Can We Learn from Our Experience and Abroad?

These lessons stand out from our experience over the years:

1. We should not depend on the market to take the lead in deciding what new technologies should be brought forward into health care, given this warning by the authors of the excellent 2021 book *System Error: Where Big Tech Went Wrong and How We Can Reboot:*

    If we accept that technology is simply beyond our control, we cede our future to engineers, corporate leaders, and venture capitalists. Some might pin their hopes on the market, thinking it will look out for our interests, deliver us the technologies we want, and weed out those that are not useful or might even do harm. But the market is good at some of this and not at others. It rewards profit without regard to social consequences. It prizes efficiency while ignoring other values. It celebrates domination. These priorities are encoded in the algorithms that power new technologies, the metrics that drive company strategy, and the regulatory environment that governs what companies may and may not do [19].

2. We should adopt cost-effectiveness analysis as a required way to assess new technologies.
3. We should evaluate new technologies concerning their cost-benefits to both individuals and populations.
4. We should depend on science, physician leadership, and responsible government to take the lead on what new medical technologies should be adopted. The Office of Technology Assessment (or a renamed agency for similar responsibilities) should be re-established and well-funded as a key part of the evaluation process.
5. Without that kind of process, proposals for new technologies should not be put up for debate and decision in Congress, as the above authors of *System Error* observe:

> *Despite our enthusiasm for the role of democracy in governing technology, our democratic institutions do not always inspire much hope. There have been far too many moments when politicians have demonstrated their ignorance of how new technologies work. We have watched parties on both the left and right curry favor with leading tech companies, cognizant of their market power and political influence. And the polarization and legislative gridlock in so many democratic societies make it difficult—if not impossible—to have reasoned discussions about how to balance competing values [20].*

6. We can learn from the positive experience of other countries' health care systems.
7. Ongoing evaluation of new technologies in use should guide their continuance.

Conclusion

Here again, at the end of this third chapter, we have seen unrelenting forces that increase costs and prices of health care in this country—primarily through corporate stakeholders in the medical-industrial complex, the private health insurance industry, and medical technologies themselves. In each case, the story is the same— no effective cost containment in sight. Industry and their lobbyists continue to oppose cost-effective analysis as a key part of evaluating new medical technologies. That is especially ironic since other countries have since effectively modeled their own medical technology assessment agencies after our original Office of Technology, which we shut down in 1995 [21]. In the next chapter, instead of dealing with this dilemma, we will find more ways that this pattern continues inexorably.

References

[1] Deyo, RA, Patrick, DL. *Hope or Hype: The Obsession with Medical Advances and the High Cost of False Promises*. New York. *AMACOM*, 2005, p.6.
[2] Ibid # 1, p. 60.
[3] Ornstein, C, Weber, T, Jones, RG. We found over 700 doctors who were paid more than a million dollars by drug and medical device companies. *ProPublica*, October 17, 2019.
[4] Serafini, M, Barrett, R. Secret deals drive higher prescription drug costs. *Tarbell*, May 24, 2018.
[5] Tahir, D. Heartbeat-tracking technology raises patients' and doctors' worries. *Kaiser Health News*, April 20, 2022.
[6] Emett, A. A Big PhRMA raises price of cancer drug by 1,400 percent. *Nation of Change*, December 27, 2016.
[7] Martyn, A. States are trying to cap the price of insulin. Pharmaceutical companies are pushing back. *FairWarning*, August 16, 2020.
[8] Silverman, S. ICER says price hikes on 7 drugs were made without proof of new benefits, costing the U.S. 5.1 billion. *STAT*, October 8, 2019.
[9] Ibid # 1, p. 259.
[10] Cavazzoni, P. *FDA's decision to approve new treatment for Alzheimer's disease*. FDA Center for Drug Evaluation and Research, FDA News Release, June 7, 2021.
[11] Walker, J. Medicare won't cover new Alzheimer's drug. *Wall Street Journal*, April 8, 2022: A 3.
[12] Demko, P. Healthcare's hired hands: When the stakes rise in Washington, healthcare interests seek well-connected lobbying firms. *Modern Healthcare*, October 6, 2014.
[13] Saluja, Sonali, Steffie Woolhandler, David U Himmelstein, David Bor, Danny McCormick. Unsafe drugs were prescribed more than one hundred million times in the United States before being recalled. *Intl J Health Services*, June 14, 2016.
[14] Feigal, DW, Gardner, SN, McClennan, J. Ensuring safe and effective medical devices. *N Engl J Med* 348: 191, 2003.
[15] Meier, B. Hip implants U.S. rejected sold overseas. *New York Times*, February 12, 2012: A1.
[16] Thomas, L. *The Fragile Species*. New York. *Macmillan*, 1992, pp. 10-15.
[17] Lagnado, L. When a medical test leads to another, and another. *Wall Street Journal*, August 20, 2016: D 1.
[18] Fisher, ES, Welch, HG. Avoiding the unintended costs of growth in medical care: How might more be worse? *JAMA* 281: 446-453, 1999.

[19] Reich, R, Sahami, M, Weinstein, JM. *System Error: Where Big Tech Went Wrong and How We Can Reboot*. New York. *Harper Collins Publishers*, 2021, p. xxxi.
[20] Ibid # 18, pp. 257-258.
[21] Ibid # 1, p. 271.

Chapter 4

Increasing Privatization, Profiteering and Corruption

> *Our health care system has been driven largely by profit, rather than by measures of health. Countless providers, companies, consultants and intermediaries are trying to get their piece of the $3.5 trillion pie that is U.S. health care. In 21st century health care, everything is revenue, and so everything is billed* [1].
>
> —Dr. Elisabeth Rosenthal, ER physician, editor-in-chief of Kaiser Health News, and author of *An American Sickness: How Healthcare Became Big Business and How You Can Take It Back.*

As we saw in the last chapter, new medical technologies over the last 50 years have led to inexorable increases in prices and costs of health care. Here, we examine three other major areas that have produced the same result with often negative impacts on affordability and access to care.

1. Increasing Privatization

Medicine and health care have been transformed over the last 50 years from a public good to a private good, as shown by Donald Cohen and Allen Mikaelian in their recent book, *The Privatization of Everything: How the Plunder of Public Goods Transformed America and How We Can Fight Back.* As they say:

> *Every time a politician hands public health care programs over to private-sector profiteering, it creates a greater burden on those least able to afford it. The obvious result is a group of people who are sicker and poorer, so it's convenient for politicians to do this in the name of the free market, efficiency, and consumerism. It absolves them* [2].

A brief excursion around the medical-industrial complex is instructive in showing how widely privatization has impacted the delivery of U.S. health care service with ever-increasing costs. These markers tell the story of relentless privatization of health care:

1.1. Hospitals

- Merging into large consolidated hospital systems, reaching near monopoly levels, then charging what the traffic will bear [3].

1.2. Ambulance Services

- Since two of the three largest air ambulance companies were bought up by private equity firms, costs of flights have soared, with some 80 percent of which not being emergencies [4]. Some bills are astronomical and not readily explained, such as one for $489,000 for an air ambulance flight from Colorado to North Carolina and ground transport between the hospitals and airports [5].

1.3. Nursing Homes

- The Carlyle Group bought ManorCare, the second largest nursing home chain in the country, then cut staff, was cited for health code violations and harm to patients, and filed for bankruptcy [6].

1.4. Pharmaceutical Industry

- Secret deals made with drug makers and pharmacy benefit managers, such as CVS Caremark and Express Scripts, drive higher prices for prescription drugs, then further increased through corporate mergers [7].

1.5. Private Health Insurers

- Privatized Medicare plans game the system through high overpayments from the government, restrict choice through narrowed networks, and deny 18 percent of claims [8].
- Privatized Medicaid plans often outsource their work of "coordinating" enrollees' care to subcontractors (that may be owned by private equity firms), who make money by denying or skimping on services [9].

1.6. Jails

- Death rates in U.S. jails were 18-58 percent higher from 2008 to 2019 in jails with health care managed by private companies compared to those with publicly managed care [10].

Many studies have documented that investor-owned facilities of many kinds, when compared to their not-for-profit counterparts, have consistently led to higher costs of care with lower quality. See Table 1.1 [11-25].

2. Profiteering across the Medical-Industrial Complex

Private equity requires special attention when it comes to widespread profiteering detrimental to every facility or segment of the health care system that it impacts because of its planned buy and sell practice. This is how a 2020 in-depth report by the Center for Economic and Policy Research describes its broad reach:

> *Private equity firms began buying out hospitals and nursing homes in the 2000s before moving into the more lucrative niches post-2010—ambulatory surgery, radiology, anesthesiology, emergency room management, neo-natal units, burn clinics, and trauma units, IT health and bill collecting. More recently, they have moved into nonhospital-based physician specialties—dermatology, dental practice management, case management, ophthalmology, and orthopedics—as well as behavioral health [22].*

Here are specific examples of profiteering across a wide sweep of the health care system:

2.1. Hospitals

- Charging double or even triple what Medicare will pay [23].
- REIT private equity takeovers leading to closures after profits [24].

2.2. Physician Owned Facilities

- Physician owners of specialty hospitals and ambulatory surgery centers have conflicts of interest which maximize their revenues by charging for their own services, sharing in a facility profit, and increasing the value of their investment in order to get around anti-kickback regulations. Physician owners of CT and other imaging centers have been found to order two to eight times as many imaging procedures as those who do not own such equipment, for an estimated $40 billion a year worth of unnecessary imaging each year [25].

2.3. Purchase of Physicians' Practices

- Venture capitalists through private equity firms have targeted physicians' practices in several specialties as a way to seek maximal investor return, usually over a 3 to 5-year period. The usual strategy is to pressure the physicians to see more patients, perform more procedures, and increase revenues. Before selling the practices, the new owners then typically load the practices with excessive debt in order to raise the likelihood of default and bankruptcy as a profit-taking strategy. Target specialties to date have included dermatology [26], ophthalmology [27], and obstetrics-gynecology [28].

2.4. Private Health Insurance

- Private health insurers up-code billing codes for which claims are made without care being provided [29].

Table 4.1. HMO "House calls": A new upcoding scam

- HMOs send its "housecall" doctor – or one from Mobile Medical Examination Services Inc.
- Doctor seeks out unimportant diagnoses, e.g. mild arthritis
- No treatment offered
- Extra diagnoses allow HMOs to upcode - adding > $3 billion/yr to Medicare Advantage payments
- Efforts to outlaw upcoding "housecalls" were scrapped after industry lobbying blitz

Source: Schulte, Center for Public Integrity, 2014.

- Lobbying the government for continuation of some $685 billion a year in subsidies, which the CBO projects will double in another 10 years [30, 31].

2.5. PhRMA

- Big pharmacy chains profiting from the opioid epidemic by ordering huge quantities of prescription opioid pills.
- COVID vaccine profiteering [32] As a complete departure from Jonas Salk's conviction that the new polio vaccine he developed in 1955 should be for the people and not for making a personal fortune [33], Pfizer and Moderna received government contracts of $1.95 billion and almost $1 billion, respectively, for development of their COVID vaccines, and then will likely make a profit margin between 60 and 80 percent because of their receipt of public money, not their own investment [34].
- Pfizer and Astellas marketing Xtandi, their break-through drug for prostate cancer for $189,800 a year, after having received substantial federal funding for its development and raising its price by 90 percent over the last 8 years [35].

3. Corruption, Even Fraud

- Doctor-owned testing clinics, such as Comprehensive Pain Specialists for detection of opioid drugs, charging high billings to Medicare and other payers [36].
- Hospitals paying high kickbacks to employed physicians in return for their bringing more referrals, paying some as if they are full-time or paying them up to four times what their peers earn [37].
- Nursing homes, after purchase by private equity firms, discharging or evicting patients when they become sicker and need more care [38].
- Overbilling Medicare and the Federal Employees Health Benefits Program for medically unnecessary rehabilitation services, as Guardian Elder Care Holdings did while operating more than 50 nursing facilities in three states [39].
- As home health care has become a big industry, various fraudulent practices have been taken up by some home health agencies, including billing for false work; falsifying patients' diagnoses as needs for care; and discharging patients and then re-admitting them without a change in the patient's medical condition [40, 41].
- Two-thirds of the nation's hospices are now for-profit, whereby they provide fewer services, have less clinically skilled staff, more discharges of sicker patients and more hospital and emergency department use [42]. As one example of fraud, state auditors found that hospices in Los Angeles County likely overbilled Medicare by $105 million in 2019 alone [43].
- Medical billing fraud, estimated to account for about $270 billion a year [44].

In his landmark book, *License to Steal: How Fraud Bleeds America's Health Care System,* Malcolm Sparrow, Professor of the Practice of Public Management at Harvard University's John F. Kennedy School of Government, estimated in 2000 that fraud accounted for $350 billion a year. As he said at the time:

> *Health care fraud remains uncontrolled, and mostly invisible. For Americans, this problem represents one of the most massive and persistent fiscal control failures in their history. Many who work the system, or feed off it, like it so. For those who profit from it, health care*

fraud is not seen as a problem, but as an enormously lucrative enterprise, worth defending vigorously [45].

Conclusion

This story of profiteering and corruption, accelerated by privatization, has derailed the original intent of health care for the common good. It does not bode well for the future of health care unless major changes can be achieved in financing and incentives within this large industry. Cohen and Mikaelian, authors of *The Privatization of Everything*, give us some hope on the horizon in these words:

> *In spite of the vast amounts of power and money focused on privatizing public goods, there remain several reasons to be hopeful, and there is much that we can do. In the end, paradoxical as it seems, privatization is not just about money or about who provides what service; privatization is about values, about whether we are committed to promoting the general welfare as enshrined in the preamble to the Constitution, and about what we the public deem to be public goods* [46].

We will deal with what reform may be possible in Part 3 of this book, but for now we move into the next chapter to discuss the all-important matter of what kind of values will prevail then.

References

[1] Rosenthal, E. Analysis: Choosing a plan from the impossible health care maze. *Kaiser Health News*, December 6, 2019.
[2] Cohen, D, Mikaelian, A. *The Privatization of Everything: How the Plunder of Public Goods Transformed America and How We Can Fight Back*. New York. *The New Press*, 2021, 172-173.
[3] Abelson, R. When hospitals merge to save money, patients often pay more. *New York Times*, November 14, 2018.
[4] Castagno, P. How private equity exploited ambulances and vulnerable patients. *Citizen Truth*, October 3, 2019.
[5] Appleby, J. The case of the $489,000 air ambulance ride. *Kaiser Health News*, March 25, 2022.

[6] Whoriskey, P, Keating, D. Overdoses, bedsores, broken bones: What happened when a private-equity firm sought to care for society's most vulnerable? *The Washington Post*, November 25, 2018.
[7] Serafini, M, Barrett, R. Secret deals drive higher prescription drug costs. *Tarbell*, May 24, 2018.
[8] Silvers, JB. This is the most realistic path to Medicare for All. *New York Times*, October 16, 2019.
[9] Terhune, C. Coverage denied: Medicaid patients suffer as layers of private companies profit. *Kaiser Health News*, January 3, 2019.
[10] Szep, J. Dying inside: The hidden crisis in America's jails. *Reuters*, October 16, 2020.
[11] Silverman, EM, Skinner, JS, & Fisher, ES. The association between for-profit hospital ownership and increased Medicare spending. *N Engl J Med* 341: 420, 1999.
[12] Woolhandler, S, Himmelstein, DU. Costs of care and administration at for-profit and other hospitals in the United States. *N Engl J Med* 36: 769, 1997.
[13] Ivory, D, Protess, B, Daniel, J. When you dial 911 and Wall Street answers. *New York Times*, June 25, 2016.
[14] Himmelstein, David U, Steffie Woolhandler, Ida Hellander, Sidney M Wolfe. Quality of care in investor-owned vs not-for-profit HMOs. *JAMA* 282: 159, 1999.
[15] Harrington, Charlene, Steffie Woolhandler, Joseph Mullan, Helen Carrillo and David U Himmelstein. Does investor-ownership of nursing homes compromise the quality of care? *Am J Public Health* 91 (9): 1, 2001.
[16] Munoz, R. How health care insurers avoid treating mental illness. *San Diego Union Tribune*, May 22, 2002.
[17] Devereaux, PJ, Schünemann, HJ, Ravindran, N, Bhandari, M, Garg, AX, Choi, PT-L, Grant, BJB, Haines, T, Lacchetti, C, Weaver, B, Lavis, JN, Cook, DJ, Haslam, DRS, Sullivan, T, and Guyatt, GH. Comparison of mortality between for-profit and private not-for-profit hemodialysis centers: A systematic review and meta-analysis. *JAMA* 288: 2449, 2002.
[18] Garg, PP, Frick, KD, Diener-West, M, and Powe, NR. Effect of the ownership of dialysis facilities on patients' survival and referral for transplantation. *N Engl J Med* 341: 1653, 1999.
[19] Pear, R. U.S. pays billions for 'assisted living,' but what does it get? *New York Times*, February 18, 2018.
[20] Cabin, William, David U Himmelstein, Michael L Siman, Steffie Woolhandler. For profit Medicare home health agencies' costs appear higher and quality appears lower compared to not-for-profit agencies. *Health Affairs* 33 (8): 1460-1465, 2014.
[21] Waldman, P. Preparing Americans for death lets hospices neglect end of life. *Bloomberg*, July 22, 2011.
[22] Appelbaum, E, Batt, R. Private equity buyouts in healthcare: Who wins, who loses? Working paper no. 118, *Center for Economic and Policy Research*, March 15, 2020.
[23] Abelson, R. Many hospitals charge double or even triple what Medicare would pay. *New York Times*, May 9, 2019.
[24] Spegele, B. Small firm bet big on hospital property. *Wall Street Journal*, February 15, 2022.

[25] Bach, P. Paying doctors to ignore patients. *New York Times*, July 24, 2008.
[26] Meyer, H. Concerns grow as private equity buys up dermatology practices. *Modern Healthcare*, July 24, 2017.
[27] O'Donnell, Eloise May, Gary Joseph Lelli, Sami Bhidya, Lawrence P Casalino. The growth of private equity investment in health care: Perspectives from ophthalmology. *Health Affairs* 39 (6): June 2020.
[28] Bruch, JD, Borsa, A, Song, Z, and Richardson, SS. Expansion of private equity involvement in women's health care. *JAMA Internal Medicine*, August 24, 2020.
[29] Schulte, F, Donald, D. Cracking the codes: How doctors and hospitals have collected billions in questionable Medicare fees. *Center for Public Integrity*, May 19, 2014.
[30] Ockerman, E. It costs $685 billion a year to subsidize U.S. health insurance. *Bloomberg News*, May 23, 2018.
[31] Potter, W. Take it from me, tweaks won't fix health care. *USA Today*, December 14, 2018.
[32] Abelson, Jenn, Aaron Williams, Andrew Ba Tran, Meryl Kornfield. At height of crisis, Walgreens handled nearly one in five of the most addictive opioids. *The Washington Post*, November 7, 2019.
[33] Smith, J. *Patenting the sun: Polio and the Salk vaccine*. New York. *William Morrow*, 1990, p. 159.
[34] Hiltzik, M. Private firms keep stranglehold on COVID vaccines, though you paid for the research. *Los Angeles Times*, November 16, 2020.
[35] Hiltzik, M. U.S. could slash a cancer drugs price. *Los Angeles Times*, February 17, 2022.
[36] Schulte, F, Lucas, E. Liquid gold: Pain doctors soak up profits by screening urine for drugs. *Kaiser Health News*, November 6, 2017.
[37] Rau, K. Hospitals accused of paying doctors large kickbacks in quest for patients. *Kaiser Health News*, May 31, 2019.
[38] Ibid # 5.
[39] Guardian Elder Care to pay $15.4 million to settle False Claims Act charges. *Corporate Crime Reporter* 34 (8): February 24, 2020.
[40] Confessore, N, Kershaw, N. As home health industry booms, little oversight to counter fraud. *New York Times*, September 2, 2007.
[41] Lee, SC. Assistant United States Attorney (ND-IL) Law enforcement observations about home-health fraud, 2020.
[42] Aldridge, MD. Hospice tax status and ownership matters for patients and families. *JAMA Internal Medicine*, August 21, 2021.
[43] Poston, B, Christensen, K. Fraud is found in hospice system. *Los Angeles Times*, March 30, 2022.
[44] Estimate by Professor Malcolm Sparrow; personal communication from Ralph Nader, January 30, 2021.
[45] Sparrow, MK. *License to Steal: How Fraud Bleeds America's Health Care System*. Boulder, CO. *Westview Press*, 2000, p. xvii.
[46] Ibid # 2, p. 17.

Chapter 5

Change of Values from a Service Ethic to a Business "Ethic"

> *The essence of medicine is so different from that of ordinary business that they are inherently at odds. Business concepts of good management may be useful in medical practice, but only to a degree. The fundamental ethos of medical practice contrasts sharply with that of ordinary commerce, and market principles do not apply to the relationship between physician and patient. Such insights have not stopped the growing domination of market ideology over medical professionalism* [1].
>
> —Arnold Relman, M.D., nephrologist, editor of *The New England Journal of Medicine* (1977 to 1991), long-time advocate for physicians to retain an ethical commitment to patients and society

> *The low level which commercial morality has reached in America is deplorable. We have humble God rearing Christian men among us who will stoop to do things for a million dollars that they ought not to be willing to do for less than 2 millions* [2].
>
> —Mark Twain, 1902

In an address to the New York Academy of Medicine 32 years ago, Dr. Edmund Pellegrino, physician, ethicist, founder and director of Georgetown University's Center for the Advanced Study of Ethics, pointed out the central dilemma facing the medical profession was to make a choice between two opposing moral orders—one based on the primacy of our ethical obligations to the sick, the other to the primacy of self-interest and the marketplace" [3]. That central dilemma is still with us, though to a considerable extent the decision has been made for the profession by the changes described in preceding chapters about the corporate controlled health care marketplace. The goals of this chapter are (1) to briefly describe the traditional service ethic in health care; (2) to show how it has been largely replaced by a business "ethic" to maximize revenues at the expense of patients; and (3) to consider the adverse impacts of these changes on physicians, other health professionals and patients.

1. Traditional Service Ethic of Health Care

Physicians have held the public trust, for the most part, of being in a morally-drive profession since the time of Hippocrates in Greece (460-377 B.C.) [4]. Graduates of most medical schools, as they join the medical community, "pro-fess" through the Hippocratic oath that they will uphold service above self-interest and embrace such virtues as honesty, compassion, and fidelity to trust [5].

The practice of medicine in the 1950s was mostly a cottage industry with physicians self-employed in small independent group practice, even solo practice. Since then, as shown in preceding chapters, health care has been transformed by a for-profit medical-industrial complex, with a majority of physicians now employed by others, especially by hospital systems. Their employers have placed maximizing of profits above service to patients, with physicians often unable to intervene on behalf of their patients.

The independent, non-profit and non-partisan Hastings Bioethics Research Institute, in its 1996 Report on the Goals of Medicine, foresaw the hazards of a free-wheeling medical marketplace in these terms:

> *Everything can be bought and sold, turned into a commodity. But some goods, values and institutions can too easily be corrupted by commodification. Health is a vital human good, and medicine a basic way of promoting it. Commercializing them, even for the sake of choice and efficiency, runs a potent risk of subverting them. The integrity of medicine itself is at stake. An excessive and unbalanced commercialization and privatization of medicine is a dire threat to the very goals of medicine* [6].

Some medical organizations have attempted to fight back against these changes. A Charter on Medical Professionalism was developed by the American Board of Internal Medicine Foundation, the American College of Medicine-American Society of Internal Medicine Foundation, and the European Federation of Internal Medicine. In 2002, it identified three fundamental principles that should underpin medical professionalism (Table 5.1) [7].

Table 5.1. Fundamental principles of medical professionalism

Principle of primacy of patient welfare. This principle is based on a dedication to serving the interest of the patient. Altruism contributes to the trust that is central to the physician-patient relationship. Market forces, societal pressures, and administrative exigencies must not compromise this principle.

Principle of patient autonomy. Physicians must have respect for patient autonomy. Physicians must be honest with their patients and empower them to make informed decisions about their treatment. Patients' decisions about their care must be paramount, as long as those decisions are in keeping with ethical practice and do not lead to demands for inappropriate care.

Principle of social justice. The medical profession must promote justice in the health care system, including the fair distribution of health care resources. Physicians should work actively to eliminate discrimination in health care, whether based on race, gender, socioeconomic status, ethnicity, religion, or any other social category.

Source: Project of the ABIM Foundation. ACP-ASIM Foundation and European Federation of Internal Medicine. Medical professionalism in the new millennium: A physician charter. *Ann Intern Med* 136(3):244, 2002.

Unfortunately, however, these fine aspirational goals have done little to reverse or even influence the relentless corporate transformation of U.S. health care.

2. The Dominant Business "Ethic" of Today's Health Care Marketplace

Physicians, together with other health professionals in today's corporate controlled marketplace, have become classified as "providers," as noted by Dr. Bill Phillips, Professor Emeritus of Family Medicine at the University of Washington and past editor of the *Annals of Family Medicine*:

> *I believe the term "provider" is a strategic weapon in the commercial war to commoditize medical professionals and health care. A provider is more impersonal than a doctor, nurse or counselor. The*

impersonal becomes the interchangeable. Provider contracts are more manageable than caring relationships [8].

Today, the corporate-controlled health care marketplace constitutes more than one-sixth of the nation's economy, and has left the traditional service ethic far behind, as these markers illustrate:

- 70 percent of U.S. physicians now work for corporate employers, especially hospital systems, under pressure to maximize revenues for their employers [9].
- Private equity firms buying hospitals, then cutting staff, reducing quality of care, loading them with debt, and finally selling them at a profit as many are forced into bankruptcy [10]. A similar approach has been taken for nursing homes [11] and physician practices ranging from emergency care [12] and obstetrics-gynecology [13] to mental health services [14].
- Private equity firms are also moving into primary care for increased profits and control of the system, especially in pharmacy-based clinics [15].
- Subversion of the electronic health record from its original goal to exchange medical and health care information to a billing instrument whereby physicians are pressured by their employers to up-code diagnoses for which care was not provided [16].
- Privatized Medicare Advantage gaming the system through overpayments and overstating the severity of patients' illnesses [17]; The Centers of Medicaid and Medicare Services even promoting Medicare Advantage as full replacement for traditional Medicare [18].
- Privatized Medicaid managed care raising revenues through such means as falsifying new enrollee registrations, disenrolling sicker patients, or even embezzlement of capitation funds paid by states [19].
- Price gouging by pharmaceutical companies that knows no bounds; two examples—Mylan's EpiPen,
emergency allergic reactions, increased its price by more than six-fold over several years [20], and Aduhelm, Biogen's new Alzheimer's drug, setting its initial annual price at $56,000 even when its efficacy was not yet proven [21].

- Supposedly not-for-profit hospitals avoiding charitable care as required by law for patients with incomes below twice the federal poverty level, then sending them to collection agencies for non-payment [22].
- Big PhRMA carrying out direct-to-consumer drug advertising, banned in many other countries, often with deception and disinformation [23].
- Investor-owned care, consistently resulting in higher costs and lower quality of care (Table 1.1) [24].
- Employer-sponsored health insurance, previously the backbone of the insurance industry, has become increasingly unaffordable for both employers and employees [25].
- The average denial rate for in-network claims through the Affordable Care Act's marketplace plans is 17 percent as insurers game the system to maximize profit [26].

The dissemination of medical information has recently become a growing industry of its own, already rife with profiteering, as exemplified by Outcome Health, a digital provider of medical information and advertising for physicians' offices and pharmaceutical companies; it defrauded its clients by misrepresenting the quality and quantity of its advertising services [27]. Another new venture, Graphite Health, is starting a pilot project to develop a platform to enable app developers to abstract and standardize health system data, and then to create an open and secure online marketplace for digital tools that providers can access [28]. Ries Robinson, its CEO, has advanced, to his credit, the embrace of a digital Hippocratic oath for all decisions for the extended medical community using its platform [29]. That would require trust, however, at a level not justified based on history and the above pervasive questionable practices.

3. Adverse Impacts on the Medical Profession and Health Professionals

Unfortunately, as preceding chapters have shown, the medical profession has lost out in so many ways since corporate control of our market-based "system" has taken center stage. Despite its long tradition of service, the practice of medicine in the U.S., has been enveloped by the corporate profit-driven business "ethic" at a high cost to physicians. Their independent practices have all but disappeared while they have become burdened with EHR/deskwork for more than 14 hours per week (Figure 1.1) and surrounded by hordes of managers (Figure 1.2). The quality and continuity of the physician-patient relationship has been distorted by profit-taking by their employers, all the while at a loss of their clinical autonomy.

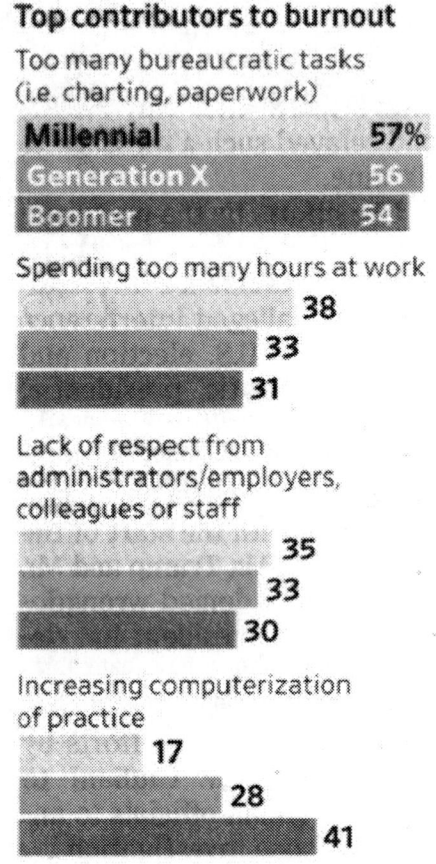

Source: National Academy of Medicine, Washington D.C., 2017.

Figure 5.1. Burnout strikes mid-career physicians hard.

A 2017 report found that more than one-half of U.S. physicians are exhibiting signs of burnout, together with emotional exhaustion and a decreased sense of personal accomplishment [30]. A more recent study of

15,000 mid-career physicians found that almost one-half of those between ages 40 and 54 were feeling burned out (Figure 5.1) [31].

Dr. Gayle Stephens, well known family physician, leader, moral philosopher and author of *The Intellectual Basis of Family Practice*, had this to say more than 30 years ago about public service being a key foundation of medical professionalism:

> *If physicians lose the compulsion for public service, they will also lose the protection and prerogatives for self-discipline and professional autonomy that the medical profession has enjoyed for centuries. There is no doubt that these have already been seriously eroded, but the way to repair the damage is by convincing the public that physicians intend to be responsible for the public's well-being, and will use their power and influence to protect the weak and the sick who are at the bottom of the ladder of privilege* [32].

Rosemary Stevens, Professor of History and Sociology of Science at the University of Pennsylvania for many years, has recommended these fundamental issues for the profession to address regardless of who controls health care:

1. "The ability to treat patients, using high standards of care, without undue concerns about cost and insurance issues as these affect individual patients.
2. Satisfaction in providing continuity of care to patients.
3. Building and maintaining trusting relationships with patients and with the general public.
4. Opportunities to participate creatively in improving the network or system on behalf of patients.
5. Good information systems for more effective patient care and continuous improvement in clinical and team skills.
6. The ability to exercise professional curiosity (most formally, through clinical research and evaluation).
7. Open and fair communications with other members of the health care organization, including managers.
8. Reasonable working conditions and income levels" [33].

Conclusion

Is there any light at the end of the tunnel for the medical profession? There may be, as we will see in Part 3 of this book. Along the way, we need to consider these four questions, still mostly unanswered:

1. Is health care a human right or a privilege based on ability to pay?
2. Who is the health care system for, profiteering corporate stakeholders, their shareholders and Wall Street investors, or patients, families and taxpayers?
3. Should health care be just another commodity for sale in a largely for-profit market-based system, or essential services based on medical necessity?
4. What ethic should prevail in health care, a business "ethic" maximizing revenue to providers, or a service ethic based on needs of patients and their families? [34]

For now, however, we turn to further describing the shortfalls of the current medical marketplace in Part 2 as the basis for required reform of our non-system.

References

[1] Relman, AS. The new medical-industrial complex. *N Engl J Med* 303: 969-970, 1980.
[2] Ayres, A (ed.) *The Wit and Wisdom of Mark Twain.* New York: *Meridian Books,* 12987, p. 31.
[3] Pellegrino, ED. The medical profession as a moral community. Bulletin. *Bull NY Acad Med* 66 (3): 221, 1990.
[4] Pellegrino, ED. The Hippocratic Oath and clinical ethics. *J. Clin Ethics.* 1 (4):290-291, 1990.
[5] Edelstein, L. The professional ethics of the Greek physician. *In Ancient Medicine: Selected Papers of Ludwig Edelstein,* edited by O. Temkin & C. L. Temkin. Baltimore. *Johns Hopkins Press,* 1967, pp. 3-64.
[6] Project Report. *The Goals of Medicine: Setting New Priorities.* Hastings Center Report, November-December, 1996, p. S-20-21.
[7] Project of the ABIM Foundation. ACP-ASIM Foundation and European Federation of Internal Medicine. Medical professionalism in the new millennium: A physician charter. *Ann Intern Med* 136 (3): 244, 2002.

[8] Phillips, WR. Watching our words. *Washington Family Physician*, Spring 2021, p. 12.
[9] Physicians Advocacy Institute, as reported in *Daily Briefing, Why investors are pouring billions into primary care*. Advisory Board, a division of Optum, a wholly owned subsidiary of United Health Group. February 24, 2022.
[10] Appelbaum, E. The PR campaign to hide the real cause of those sky-high surprise medical bills. *CounterPunch*, October 18, 2019.
[11] Whoriskey, P, Keating, D. Overdoses, bedsores, broken bones: What happened when a private-equity firm sought to care for society's most vulnerable? *The Washington Post*, November 25, 2018.
[12] Arnsdorf, I. How rich investors, not doctors, profit from marking up ER bills. *ProPublica*, June 12, 2020.
[13] Bruch, Joseph D., Alexander Borsa, Zirui Song, Sarah S. Richardson. Expansion of private equity involvement in women's health care. *JAMA Internal Medicine*, August 24, 2020.
[14] Shaw, RN, Berry, OO. The rise of venture capital investing in mental health. *JAMA Psychiatry*, September 16, 2020 online.
[15] Ibid # 10.
[16] Schulte, F, Donald, D. How doctors and hospitals have collected billions in questionable Medicare fees. *Center for Public Integrity*. September 15, 2012.
[17] Walsh, MW. A whistle-blower tells of health insurers bilking Medicare. *New York Times*, May 15, 2017.
[18] Hilzik, M. Trump health plan a Trojan horse. *Los Angeles Times*, October 5, 2019.
[19] Sparrow, MK. *License to Steal: How Fraud Bleeds America's Health Care System*. Boulder, CO. *Westview Press*, 2000, pp. 71, 106-107.
[20] Court, E. Mylan's epi-pen price increases are Valeant-like in size, Shkreli-like in approach. *Marketwatch*, August 18, 2016.
[21] Walker, J, Pulliam, S. How Biogen fumbled its Alzheimer's drug. *Wall Street Journal*, January 5, 2022: A1.
[22] AG Ferguson files lawsuit against Swedish, other Providence-affiliated hospitals, for failing to make charity care accessible to thousands of Washingtonians. *Seattle Times*, February 24, 2022.
[23] Segelman, D. Unsafe drugs: Congressional silence is deadly (Part 2). *Health Letter* 18(11): 1, 2002.
[24] Geyman, JP. *America's Mighty Medical-Industrial Complex: Negative Impacts and Positive Solutions*. Friday Harbor, WA. *Copernicus Healthcare*, 2021, p. 39.
[25] Ibid # 25, p. 261-262.
[26] Pollitz, K, McDermott, D. Claims denials and appeals in ACA marketplace plans. Issue Brief. *Kaiser Family Foundation*, January 20, 2021.
[27] United States Department of Justice. Outcome Health agrees to pay $70 million to resolve fraud investigation. *Justice News*, October 13, 2019.
[28] Vaidya, A. Graphite Health launches with plans to create a marketplace for digital tools. *Health IT, Hospitals,* October 5, 2021.
[29] Robinson, R, Chopra, A. Creating a digital Hippocratic oath for the 21st century. *STAT*, February 15, 2022.

[30] Clinician well-being is essential for safe, high quality health care. *National Academy of Medicine*. Washington, D.C., 2017.
[31] Abbott, B. Burnout strikes mid-career physicians hard. *Wall Street Journal*, January 16, 2020: A3.
[32] Stephens, GG. The physician as a moral agent. *Ala J Med Sci* 16 (2): 97-108, 1979.
[33] Stevens, RA. Themes in the history of medical professionalism. *Mt Sinai J Med* 69 (6): 361.
[34] Geyman, JP. The business ethic vs. service ethic in U.S. health care: Which will prevail? *The Pharos*, Winter 2022, 40-47.

Part 2: Today's Health Care in the U.S.

> *America's health care system is neither healthy, caring, nor a system*[1].
>
> —Walter Cronkite, former editor for *CBS Evening News*

> *So, it is contrary to what we have heard rhetorically for a generation now, the individualist, greed-driven, free-market ideology is at odds with our history and with what most Americans really care about. More and more people agree that growing inequality is bad for our country, that corporations have too much power, that money in politics is corrupting democracy, and the working families and poor communities need and deserve help when the market system fails to generate shared prosperity. Indeed, the American public is committed to a set of values that almost perfectly contradicts the conservative agenda that has dominated politics for a generation now*[2].
>
> —Bill Moyers, well known journalist and political commentator and author of *Moyers on Democracy* and *Moyers on America: A Journalist and His Times*

---

[1] Cronkite, W. As quoted by Kristof, N.D. and WuDunn, S. in their book, *Tightrope: Americans Reaching for Hope*. New York. *Alfred A. Knopf*, 2020, p. 141.

[2] Moyers, B. A new story for America. *The Nation* 284 (3): 17, 2007.

Chapter 6

How Does U.S. Health Care Rank Internationally?

> *Greater reliance on individual choice and free markets are the solutions to what ails our health care system—a handful of policy changes that harness the power of markets for health services have the potential to give patients and their physicians more control over healthcare choices, create more health insurance options, lower health care costs, reduce the number of uninsured persons—and give workers a pay increase to boot* [1].
>
> —Market ideology as expressed by senior fellows at the Hoover Institution in 2006 as part of the neoliberal school of thought

> *Nothing quite exposes the inequalities that exist in American society more than the health care system. It's a complex combination of private insurance, public programs and politics that drives up costs, creating significant barriers to lifesaving medical treatment for large segments of the population. In America, access to quality health care often depends on income, employment and status* [2].
>
> —Professor Robert Hughes of Business Ethics and Legal Studies at the Wharton School of the University of Pennsylvania

Those two opening quotes, with their sharply opposing views of U.S. health care, represent an ongoing gulf of thought that is still not resolved. Similarly, there is a big difference of opinion on how U.S. health care stacks up compared to other health care systems around the world. That has been a story of two universes—one based on solid evidence, the other purveyed by believers in American exceptionalism that we have the best system in the world. This chapter has just two goals: (1) to bring together the major results of recurrent international studies by the Commonwealth Fund of 11 countries around the world; and (2) to consider some of the major reasons for our low standing internationally as a rebuttal to those convinced that U.S. health care is the best anywhere.

1. Evidence-Based Comparisons of Health Care in Eleven Countries

Figure 6.1 shows the latest overall comparisons of health care systems in 11 advanced countries. The U.S. continues to rank last, as it has for many years—an outlier in all areas of performance, except for one—care process, which includes preventive care and self-care [3].

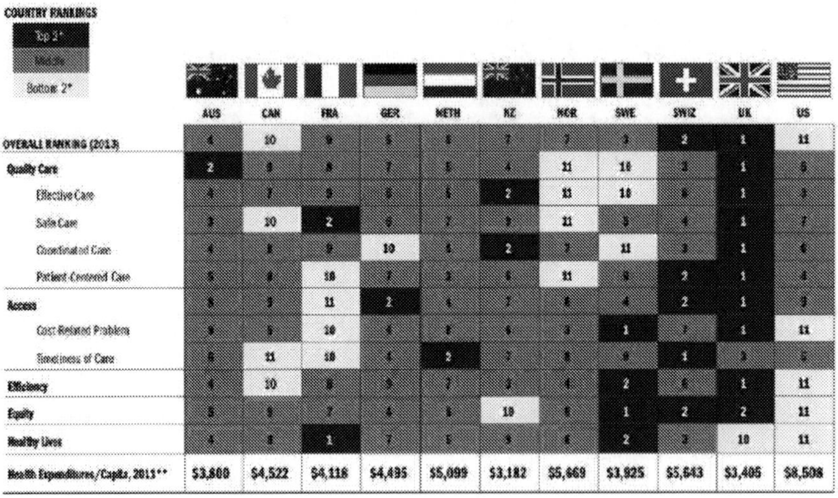

COUNTRY RANKINGS	AUS	CAN	FRA	GER	NETH	NZ	NOR	SWE	SWIZ	UK	US
OVERALL RANKING (2013)	4	10	9	5	8	7	7	3	2	1	11
Quality Care	2	9	8	7	5	4	11	10	3	1	6
Effective Care	4	7	9	8	6	2	11	10	5	1	3
Safe Care	3	10	2	6	7	9	11	5	4	1	7
Coordinated Care	4	8	9	10	5	2	7	11	3	1	6
Patient-Centered Care	5	8	10	7	3	6	11	9	2	1	4
Access	8	9	11	2	4	7	6	5	4	2	1	3
Cost-Related Problem	9	5	10	4	8	6	3	1	7	1	11
Timeliness of Care	6	11	10	4	2	7	8	9	1	3	5
Efficiency	4	10	8	9	7	3	4	2	6	1	11
Equity	5	9	7	4	8	10	6	1	2	2	11
Healthy Lives	4	8	1	7	5	9	6	2	3	10	11
Health Expenditures/Capita, 2011**	$3,800	$4,522	$4,118	$4,495	$5,099	$3,182	$5,669	$3,925	$5,643	$3,405	$8,508

Notes: *Includes ties, **Expenditures shown in $US PPP (Purchasing Power Parity). Australian $ data from 2010.

Source: Schneider, EC, Shah, A, Doty, MM et al. Mirror, Mirror 2021: Reflecting poorly. New York. *The Commonwealth Fund,* August 4, 2021, p. 3.

Figure 6.1. Overall ranking of eleven health care systems.

When it comes to equity of health care in these 11 countries, the U.S. almost falls off the chart as a stark outlier. (Figure 6.2) Australia, Germany and Switzerland rank highest on this domain, with the smallest income-related disparities [4].

The U.S. ranks last for health care outcomes, with the highest infant mortality rate (5.7 deaths per 1,000 live births), preventable mortality (177 deaths per 100,000 population), and maternal mortality (17.4 deaths per 100,000 live births). Figure 6.3 shows how the U.S. has done the least among these 11 countries in reducing avoidable mortality over the last 10 years [5].

How Does the U.S. Health Care Rank Internationally? 59

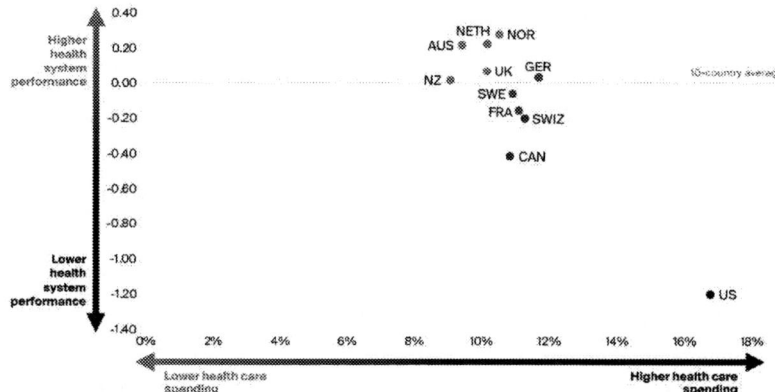

Note: Health care spending as a percent of GDP. Performance scores are based on standard deviation calculated from the 10-country average that excludes the US. See How We Conducted This Study for more detail.

Data: Spending data are from OECD for the year 2019 (updated in July 2021).

Source: Eric C. Schnelder et al., Mirror, Mirror 2021 - Reflecting Poorly: Health Care In the U.S. Compared to Other High-Income Countries (*Commonwealth Fund*, Aug. 2021). https://doi.org/10.26099.

Figure 6.2. Performance compared to health care spending.

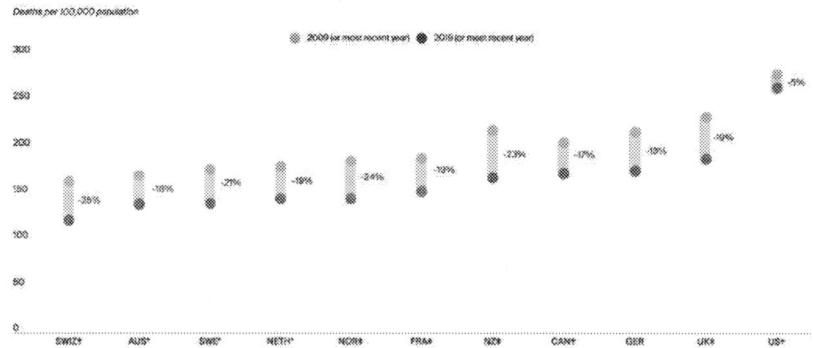

Notes: Health status: avoidable mortality. Data years are: 2009 and 2019 (Germany); 2008 and 2018 (Australia, the Netherlands, Sweden); 2007 and 2017 (Canada, Switzerland, US); and* 2006 and 2016 (France, New Zealand, Norway, UK).

Data: Commonwealth Fund analysis of data from OECD Health Statistics, July 2021.

Source: Eric C. Schneider et al., Mirror, Mirror 2021 - Reflecting Poorly: Health Care in theU.S. Compared to Other High-Income Countries (*Commonwealth Fund*, Aug. 2021). https://doLorg/10.26099/01DV-H208.

Figure 6.3. Cross national comparison of avoidable deaths.

At the end of its 2021 report, the Commonwealth Fund drew these overall conclusions. "Four features distinguish top performing countries from the United States:

1. They provide for universal coverage and remove cost barriers;
2. They invest in primary care systems to ensure that high-value services are equitably available in all communities to all people;
3. They reduce administrative burdens that divert time, efforts, and spending from health improvement efforts; and
4. They invest in social services, especially for children and working-age adults" [6].

The Commonwealth Fund also concluded that:

U.S. seniors are sicker, more economically vulnerable, and face greater financial barriers to medical care and social care than older adults in the 10 other countries [7]; and that:

The U.S. health system delivers too little of the care that's most needed—and it delivers it too late—especially for people with complex chronic illness, mental health problems, or substance abuse disorders, many of whom have faced a lifetime of inequitable access to care [8].

2. Why U.S. Rankings Are so Low

These poor results from international rankings are predictable when we consider these systemic problems of U.S. health care:

1. The U.S. still has a polyglot of public-private financing for health care that has been dysfunctional for many years. The multi-payer private insurance industry has many ways to profiteer on the backs of vulnerable Americans becoming sick or disabled. Despite its high overhead, waste, and profits, it receives federal subsidies of $685 billion a year, which the Congressional Budget Office expects to double in another ten years [9]. Figure 6.4 shows how the industry's high administrative overhead compares with five other countries.

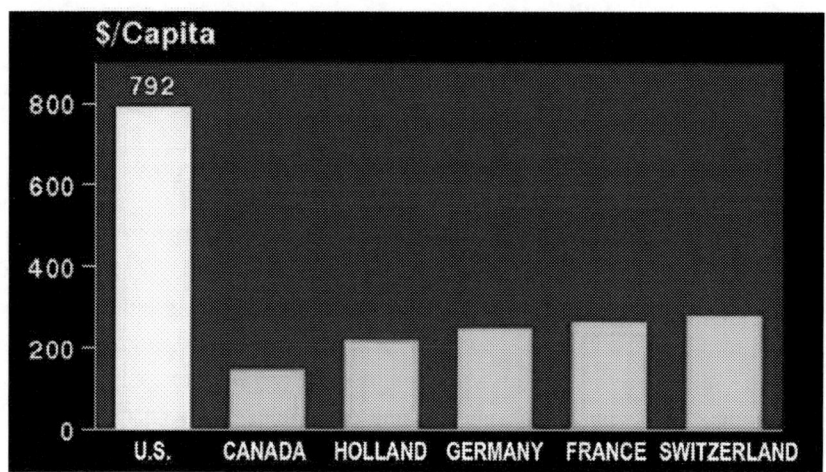

Source: OECD, 2016; NCHS; CIHI.

Figure 6.4. Insurance overhead, United States vs. five other countries, 2016.

2. The U.S. is the only country among these 11 advanced countries that does not have a solid system of guaranteed universal coverage of health care. The late Uwe Reinhardt, Ph.D., Professor of Economics and Public Affairs at Princeton University and author of the 2019 book *Priced Out: The Economic and Ethical Costs of American Health Care,* drew this conclusion:

The issue of universal coverage is not a matter of economics. Little more than 1 percent of GDP assigned to health could cover all. It is a matter of soul [10].

3. Despite the Affordable Care Act (ACA) of 2010, we still have about 30 million Americans without health insurance and another 87 million underinsured.
4. Even the insured confront barriers to access to care; as just two examples, high deductibles prevented as many as 16 million Americans with chronic conditions from seeing a physician in 2015 because of unaffordable out-of-pocket costs [11].
5. For-profit health care services and facilities, especially when investor-owned, have lower quality of care than their not-for-profit counterparts, as we saw in Chapter 1 (Table 1.1). Most facilities are

for-profit, and attempts to improve quality, such as accountable care organizations, have been ineffective [12].
6. Despite the ongoing inflation of health care prices and costs, we still have no effective cost containment on the horizon, as shown by Figures 1.4 and 1.5 in Chapter 1. As a result, one-half of U.S. adults skip necessary care because of cost compared to 12 to 15 percent of their counterparts in the UK, Norway and France [13].
7. Inequality by wealth and income has been growing exponentially for many years, to the point that the richest 1% of Americans now hold more of the nation's wealth than the bottom 90 percent of our population [14]. Those inequalities translate into persistent and increasing disparities and inequities in health care based on socioeconomic status, race/ethnicity, age, gender, and disability status.

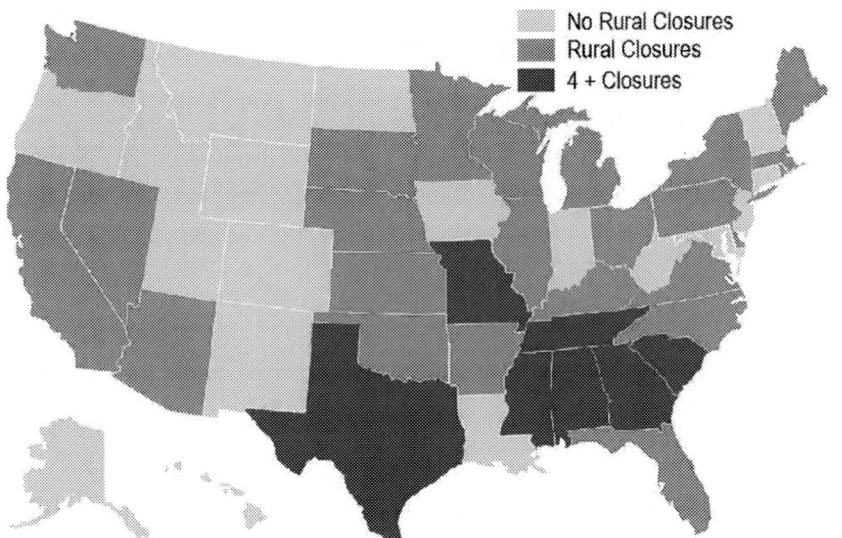

Source: Frakt, A. A sense of alarm as rural hospitals keep closing. *New York Times,* October 29, 2018.

Figure 6.5. Rural hospital closures in America since 2010.

8. Women's health care, mental health, and rural health care have been disadvantaged in the U.S. for many years. Compared to men, women are more likely to have lower wages and incomes, to be on Medicaid, and to be the primary caretakers of their children [15]. The U.S. has

a chronically underfunded, limited access system for mental health care, with many mentally ill criminalized in jail where they receive little if any care [16]. Partly as a result of under-reimbursement, rural health care has been hard hit by rural hospital closures (Figure 6.5) and shortage of health care professionals [17], leaving more than 30 million Americans more than an hour away from critical care [18].

9. Wide variations in access, equity, affordability, outcomes of care, and life expectancy have been documented by the Commonwealth Fund from one state to another [19].

10. In contrast to the other advanced countries, the U.S. has an inadequate primary care base without a policy fix yet in sight. It has been weakened by decades of underinvestment, with its growth also limited by a wide wage gap between generalists and specialists. Compared to other advanced countries, U.S. adults are the least likely to have a regular physician or place of care, or have a longstanding relationship with a primary care provider. Access to home visits or after-hours care is also lowest in the U.S. [20].

A strong system base of generalist primary care physicians trained and committed to provide first-contact, comprehensive health care is urgently needed. Today, less than 10 percent of U.S. medical graduates enter family medicine, the broadest of primary care specialties with the capacity to care for patients across the entire age spectrum. Since most medical school graduates plan to enter the highest paid medical and surgical specialties, the Association of American Medical Colleges (AAMC) predicts a shortage of between 21,000 and 55,200 primary care physicians by 2032 [21].

11. The U.S. has still not developed a federal physician workforce plan to enable increases in the numbers of residency training positions in primary care. This is in marked contrast to the United Kingdom and Canada, where goals for a generalist base of 50% and 30% primary care physicians, respectively, are well established. A logical policy fix in this country could well be to establish a goal, such as 25-30%, tied to federal support to hospitals for residency positions.

12. Public health, which is dedicated to health promotion, prevention of disease, accidents, and bad health outcomes, has been neglected and underfunded in the U.S. for many years. It is well documented that it saves more lives than individually-oriented medical care, as exemplified by the drop by one-half of age-adjusted mortality from coronary heart disease between 1950 and 1987, due more to smoking

cessation and diet than to coronary care units and cardiac bypass surgery [22, 23]. Despite its importance, however, recognition and support for public health has been declining for years, as Dr. Karen DeSalvo, when acting assistant secretary of the Department of Health and Human Services, described in 2015:

Public health infrastructure has a history of being there when necessary, but on the other hand increasingly being marginalized and underfunded year after year. We are starving our infrastructure. Even though 80 percent of people's health is influenced by what happens outside of doctors' offices and hospitals, about 97 percent of funding goes to pay for medical services [24].

13. Our free-wheeling market-based system sucks up much of the health care dollar through high prices, providing unnecessary services, its inefficiency, waste and even fraud, which collectively amounted to $765 billion a year, according to a 2013 report by the Institute of Medicine [25]. We have no reason to believe that number to be lower today.
14. Employer-sponsored health insurance, which has been the bulwark of our multi-payer financing system, is no longer affordable for employers or employees alike. In fact, as discussed in Chapter 2, it has become a barrier to urgently needed health care reform. Cost sharing through high deductibles at the point of service often results in patients delaying or foregoing necessary care as insurers mark up high profits for themselves and their shareholders [26].

Conclusion

The consistent poor showing of U.S. health care by international comparisons with other advanced countries seems certain to continue indefinitely into the future without shifting over to a public not-for-profit system of national health insurance that will ensure universal coverage for all Americans and share the risk of illness and accidents across our entire population. We will return to this subject in Chapters 9 and 13, but for now we need to move to the next chapter to consider how disparities, inequities and systemic racism stand in the way of health care justice in this country.

References

[1] Cogan, JF, Hubbard, RG, Kessler, DP. Keep government out. *Wall Street Journal*, January 13, 2006: A 12.
[2] Hughes, R. *Does the U.S. need universal health care?* Interview by Knowledge@Wharton. The Wharton School of the University of Pennsylvania, December 8, 2020.
[3] Schneider, Eric C, Arnav Shah, Michelle M Doty, Roosa Tikkanen, Katharine Fields, Reginald D Williams II. *Mirror, Mirror 2021: Reflecting poorly*. New York. *The Commonwealth Fund*, August 4, 2021, p. 3.
[4] Ibid # 3, p. 7.
[5] Ibid # 3, p. 9.
[6] Ibid # 3, p. 1.
[7] Blumenthal, D, Collins, SR, Radley, DC. 2017 Commonwealth Fund International Health Policy Survey of Older Adults in 11 Countries. New York. *The Commonwealth Fund*, December 1, 2017.
[8] Ibid # 3, p. 14.
[9] Ockerman, E. It costs $685 billion a year to subsidize U.S. health insurance. *Bloomberg News*, May 23, 2018.
[10] Reinhardt, UE. *Priced Out: The Economic and Ethical Costs of American Health Care*. Princeton, NJ. *Princeton University Press*, 2019, p. 139.
[11] The editors. Out of pocket, out of control. *Bloomberg View*, February 16, 2015.
[12] Rubin, R. How value-based Medicare payments exacerbate health care disparities. *JAMA*, February 21, 2018.
[13] Doty, Michelle M, Roosa Tikkanen, Molly Fitzgerald, Katharine Fields, Reginald D Williams II. Income-related inequalities in affordability and access to primary care in eleven high-income countries. *The Commonwealth Fund*, December 9, 2020.
[14] Hightower, J. It's time to a (teeny) tax on wealth. *The Hightower Lowdown* 21 (8): 1-2, September, 2019.
[15] Bernstein, J, Katch, H. Cutting support for economically vulnerable women is no way to celebrate Mother's Day. *The Washington Post*, May 11, 2018.
[16] Gorman, A. Use of psychiatric drugs soars in California jails. *Kaiser Health News*, May 8, 2018.
[17] Frakt, A. A sense of alarm as rural hospitals keep closing. *New York Times*, October 29, 2018.
[18] Nakajima, S. Hospital beds and the crisis of rural and underserved hospitals. *Healthcare-NOW!* 22, Summer 2020, p. 2.
[19] Radley, DC, Collins, SR, Baumgartner, JC. 2020 Scoreboard on State Health System Performance, September 2020, *The Commonwealth Fund*.
[20] Fitzgerald, M, Gunja, MZ, Tikkanen, R. Primary care in high-income countries: How the U.S. compares. New York. *The Commonwealth Fund*, March 15, 2022.
[21] Knight, V. American medical students less likely to choose to become primary care doctors. *Kaiser Health News*, July 3, 2019.

[22] Stamler, J. The marked decline in coronary heart disease mortality rates in the United States, 1968-1981: Summary of findings and possible explanations. *Cardiology* 72 (11), 1985.
[23] Goldman, L, Cook, EF. The decline in ischemic heart disease mortality rates. *Ann Intern Med* 101: 825, 1984.
[24] DeSalvo, K. As quoted by O'Donnell, J, Unger, L. Public health gets least money, but does most. *USA Today*, December 8, 2015.
[25] *Best care at Lower Cost.* Washington, D.C. *Institute of Medicine*, 2013, Table 3.1.
[26] Geyman, JP. Cost sharing for health insurance: Too big a price to pay by the insured? *CounterPunch*, February 14, 2022.

Chapter 7

Disparities, Inequities and Systemic Racism

> *American health care does a poor job of delivering health but is exquisitely designed as an inequality machine, commanding an ever-larger share of G.D.P. and funneling resources to the top of the income distribution* [1].
>
> —Angus Deaton, Ph.D., Nobel laureate in economics, Professor Emeritus of Economics and Public Affairs at Princeton University, and co-author of *Deaths by Despair and the Future of Capitalism*

As we saw in earlier chapters, the above observation by Dr. Deaton about growing inequality in U.S. health care is right on target, and has everything to do with how poorly our system does in comparison with other advanced countries. This chapter has three goals: (1) to bring brief historical perspective to disparities, inequities and racism in the U.S.; (2) to describe how they persist today in U.S. health care despite efforts to remedy them; and (3) to briefly consider new approaches that may be more effective.

1. Some Historical Perspective

1.1. Income and Wealth Disparities

The income and wealth gap between rich and poor in this country has been growing for many years, refuting the "trickle-down" theory. The Pew Research Center found that the median wealth of White households was ten times that of Black households and more than eight times that of Latinx households in 2016 ($171,000 versus $17,100 and $20,600, respectively) [2]. The richest 0.1 percent in the U.S. today control a bigger slice of the pie than at any time since 1929 [3]. Figure 7.1 shows the inexorable rise of the top 1% of our society vs. the fall of the bottom 50% since 1980, which has adverse impacts on access to affordable health care as well as housing, completion of college, and job opportunities [4]. The American Dream itself has been called into serious question by these findings.

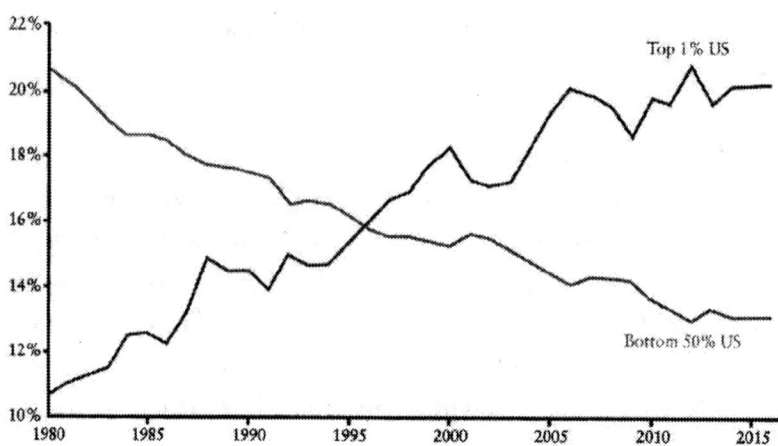

Source: Facundo Alvaredo, Lucas Chancel, Thomas Piketty, and Emmanuel Saez, *World Inequality Report* 2018 (Paris: World Inequality Lab, 2017). See https://wir2018.wid.world for data series and notes.

Figure 7.1. The rise of the top 1% and fall of the bottom 50%, 1980-2016.

Recent analyses in 2022 show an even wider gap between CEO and executive pay and median worker pay. Median pay for leaders of S & P companies rose to a record $13.4 million in 2021; for almost one-third of them, that was a raise of at least 25 percent [5]. Wall Street bonuses have soared 1,743% since 1985; if the federal minimum wage had grown at the same rate since then, it would now be $61.75 instead of $7.25 [6].

Nicholas Kristof, two-time Pulitzer Prize winning journalist and co-author of the 2020 book, *Tightrope: Americans Reaching for Hope*, calls attention to the importance of this sea change:

> *We're used to thinking of a depression as geographic, but this one is demographic. Working class Americans, often defined as those without a college degree, are caught in a dust bowl . . . It is these working Americans, white and black alike, who are seeing earnings collapse, family structure disintegrate and mortality climb. These Americans are earning less, on average, adjusted for inflation, than their counterparts back in the 1970s . . . The central fact of America today is not its economic vigor but its profound inequity* [7].

1.2. Inequities Related to Race

Disparities and inequities due to race go back some four centuries in the U.S. since the arrival of slave ships from Africa. Blacks were brought here to be owned and worked by white plantation owners, mostly in the South. At the close of the Civil War in the mid-1860s, quarantine and smallpox vaccinations were extended to soldiers of the Union Army, but not made available to Blacks [8]. In his 2012 book, *Sick from Freedom*, historian Jim Downs tells us that White leaders were afraid that free and healthy Blacks would upend the existent racial hierarchy [9]. Later medical history is stained by forced sterilizations of Black women through mass hysterectomies without consent or anesthesia and with high mortality rates in the 1880s [10].

Organized medicine failed to respond to this blatant racism. The AMA barred Black doctors, medical schools excluded Black applicants, and most hospitals and clinics segregated Black patients, so they ended up sicker and dying earlier than their White counterparts.

In response, Black communities created their own health systems and professional organizations. The National Medical Association (NMA) was organized in 1895, advocating for health care as a human right and a national plan in direct opposition to the AMA [11].

Racism has been a part of U.S. health policy since the Jim Crow era (1875-1968) in these kinds of ways:

- The GI Bill, enacted in 1944, in response to many Southern Democrats was drafted in such a way as to exclude 1.2 million Black veterans of World War II from many of its benefits, including education, home loans and insurance benefits [12].
- The 1946 Hill-Burton Act, which provided for construction of public hospitals and long-term care facilities, allowed states to construct separate and unequal facilities [13].
- The Kerr-Mills Act (1960), which provided health care to the poor, was underfunded so that few states participated, especially states having large populations of Black Americans [14].
- While Medicare and Medicaid in 1965 made important progress in reducing racial inequities in access to health care, the federal government bowed to opposition by southern states by giving them flexibility to underfund or limit Medicaid eligibility in a way that disproportionately limited coverage for racial and ethnic minority populations [15].

2. Disparities, Inequities and Racism in Today's Health Care

The corporate marketplace does not help but instead exacerbates disparities and inequities in our society. The CEO-to-worker compensation ratio has surged by more than 300 percent since 1980 [16]. Robert Reich, Professor of Public Policy at the University of California Berkeley and author of *Saving Capitalism*, adds this insight:

> *Overall, the grotesque surge in inequality that began 40 years ago is costing the median American worker $42,000 a year. The upward redistribution wasn't due to natural forces. It was contrived. As wealth accumulated at the top, so did political power to siphon off even more wealth and shaft everyone else* [17].

The U.S. population has been growing more diverse over time, with the largest growth occurring among Hispanic and Asian people. Figure 7.2 shows the current breakdown along racial lines in 2019 [18].

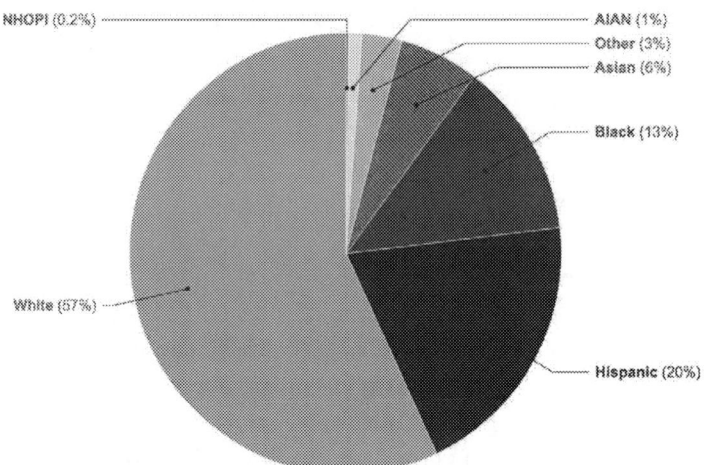

Note: Persons of Hispanic origin may be of any race but are categorized as Hispanic for this analysis; other groups are non-Hispanic. AIAN refers to American Indian and Alaska Native. NHOPI refers to Native Hawaiian and Other Pacific Islander. Other includes people with more than one race. Total may not sum to 100% due to rounding.
Source: *KFF analysis of 2019 American Community Survey, 1-Year Estimates.* • PNG.

Figure 7.2. Total United States population by race/ethnicity, 2019.

These markers of disparities, inequities and continuing racial/ethnic bias show that we still have a long way to go in this country (Figure 7.3):

- According to the Institute for Policy Studies, 49 of the 500 largest publicly traded corporate firms, with median annual CEO pay of $12.3 million, have median worker pay below the federal poverty level for a family of four [19].
- Minorities are more vulnerable than Whites to be living in poverty and to have no health insurance.
- When minority workers have employer-sponsored health insurance, they disproportionately have worse coverage, with higher premiums, cost sharing, and out-of-pocket costs [20].
- Even after adjusting for income and insurance coverage, it is well documented that Blacks and Latinos receive lower quality of care compared with Whites [21].

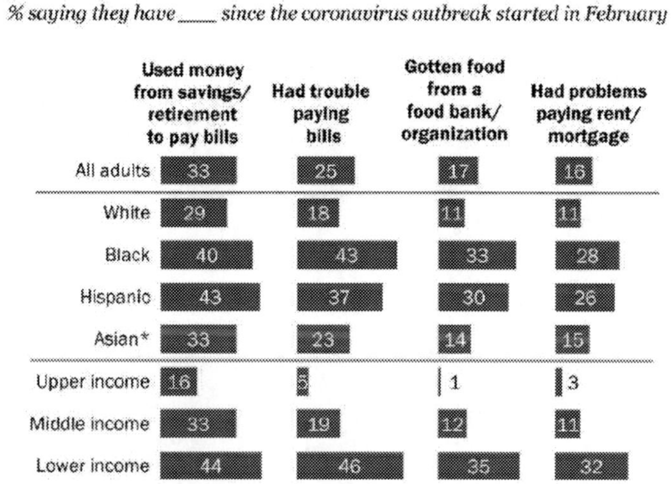

% saying they have _____ since the coronavirus outbreak started in February

	Used money from savings/ retirement to pay bills	Had trouble paying bills	Gotten food from a food bank/ organization	Had problems paying rent/ mortgage
All adults	33	25	17	16
White	29	18	11	11
Black	40	43	33	28
Hispanic	43	37	30	26
Asian*	33	23	14	15
Upper income	16	5	1	3
Middle income	33	19	12	11
Lower income	44	46	35	32

* Asian adults were interviewed in English only.

Note: White, Black and Asian adults include those who report being only one race and are not Hispanic. Hispanics are of any race. Family income tiers are based on adjusted 2019 earnings.

Source: Survey of U.S. adults conducted Aug. 3-16, 2020. "Economic Fallout from COVID-19 Continues to Hit Lower-In come Americans the Hardest" Pew Research Center.

Figure 7.3. Financial pain points during coronavirus outbreak: differ widely by race, ethnicity and income.

- A recent study of more than 240,000 nonelderly Medicaid managed care enrollees in 37 states found that, compared to White enrollees, minority enrollees had worse care experiences [22].
- Although being 12.5 percent of the U.S. population, Blacks have accounted for 23 percent of all COVID deaths [23].
- Minorities have also had a harder time than Whites during the COVID economic downturn with lower wage jobs, higher unemployment rates, and less ability to work from home.
- Figure 7.3 shows how financial pain during COVID differed by race, ethnicity and income.

Unfortunately, a majority of Americans today view systemic racism as a long-standing and continuing problem, with differences along partisan lines that may hinder rapid improvement [24] (Figure 7.4).

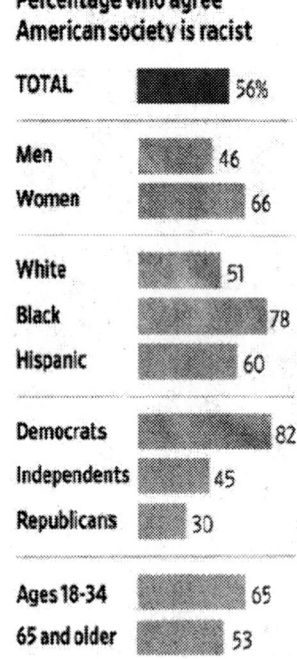

Source: *Wall Street Journal/NBC News* poll on race in America, July 2020.

Figure 7.4. Majority of Americans view our society as racist.

In their excellent 2022 article on structural racism in historical and modern U.S. health care policy, experts Ruqalljah Yearby, Brietta Clark and Jose Figueroa draw this conclusion:

> *The time has come to eradicate the structural racism in health care policy that perpetuates inequitable access to high-quality health care. If not, the racial and ethnic inequities that have occurred throughout the COVID-19 pandemic, which not only devastate minority communities but also harm the entire country, will continue. Yet this change will only come from intentional and sustained focus on addressing inequities in system reform so that health equity becomes the norm* [25].

3. What Can Be Done?

As the leaders of the National Medical Association advocated more than a century ago, the U.S., on a moral, economic and fairness basis, should finally recognize health care as a human right. All of the best performing health care systems in other advanced countries around the world came to recognize this many years ago, together with adopting one or another form of universal coverage.

It is not that we have never considered such a policy. Teddy Roosevelt, as a progressive presidential candidate in 1912, made that part of his platform, but political opposition then and at later times pushed it off the table. With the rise of the profit-driven corporate medical-industrial complex since the 1960s, neoliberalism and conservative policies have prevailed, as strengthened by Wall Street investors and corporate lobbyists. Currently, with a strong progressive caucus among Democrats in the House, universal coverage through Medicare for All waits as H. R. 1976, but again faces strong opposition among conservative Republicans.

After so many years of inaction on this important policy, we need to recall these timeless guidelines advanced by Donald Light, Ph.D., coauthor of the important 1996 book, *Benchmarks for Fairness for Health Care Reform*, whereby conservatives can support universal coverage and hold true to these four *moral* principles—*anti-free riding, personal integrity, equal opportunity, and just sharing*:

1. Everyone is covered, and everyone contributes in proportion to his or her income.

2. Decisions about all matters are open and publicly debated. Accountability of costs, quality and value of providers, suppliers, and administrators is public.
3. Contributions do not discriminate by type of illness or ability to pay.
4. Coverage does not discriminate by type of illness or ability to pay.
5. Coverage responds first to medical need and suffering.
6. Nonfinancial barriers by class, language, education, and geography are to be minimized.
7. Providers are paid fairly and equitably, taking into account their local circumstances.
8. Clinical waste is minimized through public health, self-care, prevention, strong primary care, and identification of unnecessary procedures.
9. Financial waste is minimized by simplified administrative arrangements and strong bargaining for good value.
10. Choice is maximized in a common playing field where 90-95 percent of payments go to necessary and efficient health services and only 5-10 percent to administration" [26].

Such an approach would finally bring social justice to U.S. health care and effectively address our long-standing pattern of disparities, inequities and racism. How to get there, of course, is complicated and more than challenging. The power of corporate America will have to be confronted by the unacceptable shortfalls of our existing system and the failure of our for-profit private multi-payer financing system.

Conclusion

We will address specific policy options that deal with disparities, inequities and systemic racism in Part 3 after shifting our concern to other important related areas along the way, starting next with what we can learn from how our present system has dealt with the COVID pandemic.

References

[1] Deaton, A. American health care. It's not just unfair: Inequality is a threat to our governance. *New York Times Book Review*, March 20, 2017.

[2] Brown, DA. *The Whiteness of Wealth. How the Tax System Impoverishes Black Americans—and How We Can Fix It*. New York. *Crown*, 2021, pp. 18-19.
[3] Johnson, J. World's 500 richest people gained $1.2 trillion in wealth in 2019: Analysis. *Common Dreams*, December 27, 2019.
[4] Hacker, JS, Pierson, P. *Let Then Eat Tweets: How the Right Rules in an Age of Extreme Inequality*. New York. W. and W. Norton & Company, Inc., 2020, pp. 46-47.
[5] Francis, T. CEO pay increases, heads for a new record. *Wall Street Journal*, April 4, 2022: A 1.
[6] Johnson, J. 'Jaw-dropping: Wall Street bonuses have soared 1,743% since 1985. *Common Dreams*, March 23, 2022.
[7] Kristof, ND. Part of America is still forgotten, now under Trump. *Seattle Times*, February 8, 2020.
[8] Interlandi, J. Why doesn't the United States have universal health care? The answer has everything to do with race. *New York Times*, August 14, 2019.
[9] Downs, J. *Sick from Freedom*, New York. *Oxford University Press*, 2012, pp. 78-88.
[10] Bates, L. Misogyny from the far right to the mainstream. *In the Year in Hate and Extremism 2020. Southern Poverty Law Center*. Montgomery, AL, 2021, p. 15.
[11] Ibid # 8.
[12] Blakemore, E. How the GI Bill's promise was denied to a million Black WW II veterans. *History Archive*. April 20, 2021.
[13] Yearby, R. Structural racism and health disparities: Reconfiguring the social determinants of health framework to include the root cause. *J Law Med Ethics* 48 (3): 518-526, 2020.
[14] Nolen, LT, Beckman, AL, Sandoe, E. How foundational movements in Medicaid's history reinforced rather than eliminated racial health disparities. *Health Affairs* blog, September 1, 2020.
[15] Ibid # 14.
[16] Johnson, J. As wages stagnate and executive pay 'continues to balloon,' report shows top CEOs now make 320 times more than typical worker. *Common Dreams*, August 18, 2020.
[17] Reich, R. Who gains from Trump's refusal to concede? *The Progressive Populist*, December 15, 2020, p. 13.
[18] Hill, l, Artiga, S, Haldar, S. Key facts on health and health care by race and ethnicity. *Kaiser Family Foundation*, January 26, 2022.
[19] Anderson, S, Pizzigati, S. Executive Excess 2019: Making corporations pay for big pay gaps. Institute for Policy Studies. 26th Annual Report, September, 2019.
[20] Straw, T. *Trapped by the firewall: Policy changes are needed to improve health coverage for low-income workers.* Washington, D.C., Center on Budget and Policy Priorities, December 3, 2019.
[21] Ndugga, N, Artiga, S. Disparities in health and health care: 5 key questions and answers. Issue Brief. *Kaiser Family Foundation*, May 11, 2021.

[22] Kevin H Nguyen, Ira B Wilson, Anya R Wallack, and Amal N Trivedi. Racial and ethnic disparities in patient experience of care among nonelderly Medicaid managed care enrollees. *Health Affairs* 41 (2): February, 2022.
[23] Morath, E, Omeokwe, A. Virus obliterates black job market. *Wall Street Journal*, June 10, 2020: A 1.
[24] Siddiqui, S. Majority of Americans view society as racist, poll finds. *Wall Street Journal*, July 21, 2020: A 4.
[25] Yearby, R, Brietta Clark, B, Figueroa, J. Structural racism in historical and modern U.S. health care policy. *Health Affairs* 41 (2): 187-194, February 2022.
[26] Light, DW. A conservative call for universal access to health care. *Penn Bioethics* 9 (4): 4-6, 2002.

Chapter 8

Poor System Performance during the COVID Pandemic

For too long, many Americans have held to the view that we have one of the best health care systems in the world. To the surprise of many with that view, the COVID-19 pandemic exposed long-standing problems of our system that defied that belief. This chapter has three goals: (1) to consider ways by which the U.S. was not well prepared for the COVID pandemic; (2) to describe our performance in comparison with other advanced countries; and (3) to briefly summarize lessons we can take away from that performance which can help us deal with future pandemics.

1. How the U.S. Was Ill Prepared for the Pandemic

The U.S. was less prepared than other advanced countries in coping with what arguably has been the biggest public health crisis in the nation's history, in large part because of our neglect and chronic underfunding of public health, with the serious impacts noted by Dr. Karen DiSalvo in the last chapter. An investigation reported in 2020 by the Kaiser Family Foundation and the Associated Press found that our public health infrastructure had been hollowed out before the pandemic arrived here in these kinds of ways:

- Since 2010, spending on state health departments had dropped by 16 percent per capita, and in local health departments by 18 percent, in 2019 dollars after adjusting for inflation.
- At least 38,000 state and local public health jobs had disappeared since the 2008 recession, leaving a skeletal workforce in what was once one of the world's top public health systems.
- More than three-quarters of Americans live in states that spend less than $100 per person annually on public health.

- Some public health workers earn so little that they qualify for government assistance; during the pandemic, many found themselves disrespected, ignored, or even vilified [1].

As Dr. Jonathan Oberlander, Ph.D., Professor of Social Medicine at the University of North Carolina and author of *The Political Life of Medicare,* has observed:

> *Public health is a victim of its own success. People can enjoy clean water and clear air but don't always attribute it to public health. We pay attention to public health when things go awry. But we tend to pay not a lot of attention in the normal course of events* [2].

Then arrived incoming President Donald Trump, who rapidly proceeded to set public health back more than ever before, in hard to believe ways:

- Closing of the Office for Pandemic Preparedness in the White House.
- Firing of science-based leaders who reported unwelcome news about our shortfalls of essential supplies.
- Failure to fill the National Strategic Stockpile with PPEs, N95 face masks, testing kits, and ventilators.
- Long delay to invoke the Defense Production Act, but then not using it and instead handing off to the states the responsibility to acquire their own supplies.
- That led to states fighting among themselves while even FEMA was trying to intercept their shipments for the National Stockpile!
- Rejection of help from the World Health Organization towards needed testing kits and development of a COVID vaccine while then paying nothing to the WTO for a global effort to develop and deploy diagnostics, treatments, and vaccines to deal with the pandemic [3].
- As confirmed COVID cases and deaths continued their exponential increases, Trump assigned Jared Kushner to oversee distribution of supplies from the Strategic National Stockpile, such as testing kits, personal protective equipment, and ventilators; he was later quoted as saying that "testing too many people or ordering too many ventilators would spook markets and so we just shouldn't do it" [4].

The pervasive tendency to hand over health care planning and delivery to the private sector instead of the public sector rears its head again in the case of public health, as Dr. David Blumenthal, president of the Commonwealth Fund, notes:

> *Public health is a quintessential public action. It must be done by people working together on behalf of themselves and others. In a fiercely independent culture, that is very hard to undertake . . . [While medical spending in the U.S. has skyrocketed, wariness of government helped check any parallel expansion of public health.] Americans have been much more comfortable allowing money to flow to the private sector rather than go to the public sector* [5].

2. Performance of U.S. during COVID Pandemic

The coronavirus pandemic that started in Wuhan province of China at the beginning of 2019 soon spread like wildfire around the world. Catching the U.S. off guard with our marginalized public health, our largely privatized market-based system was slow and ineffective in responding to it. Little or no response was undertaken in the first two months as the virus spread unhindered across the country. Soon all 50 states were involved as COVID-19 deaths became the leading cause of death as businesses were shuttered and employees furloughed or let go. These are some of the major impacts as the pandemic took over our country.

2.1. In the First Four Months

- At the initial epicenter, nursing homes with their high-risk patients were ill prepared for the virus. Two thirds of these facilities were in corporate chains with frequent safety violations and inadequate infection prevention.
- 3.8 million confirmed COVID-19 cases, with more than 140,000 deaths, far more than any other country in the world.
- More than 40 million Americans filing for unemployment insurance for the first time, with many of those jobs not coming back.
- Almost 27 million Americans, who became unemployed, lost their employer-sponsored health insurance due to the pandemic.

- One in four workers at high risk of serious illness if infected by the coronavirus.
- Highest unemployment rate since the Great Depression.
- Almost one-third of Americans (nearly one-half of African-Americans) having trouble paying the rent or mortgage, food, utilities, credit card bills, or medical costs [6].
- Many states confronted by budget overruns and Medicaid cuts.
- The federal budget deficit rose to $3 trillion in fiscal year 2020 [7].

2.2. One Year into the Pandemic

- With just 4 percent of the world's population, U.S. had 25% of confirmed COVID-19 cases with far more deaths and no control in sight, while our European counterparts had effectively flattened the curve of new COVID patients (Figure 8.1).
- Beset with a primary care shortage, our outpatient resources and hospitals were overrun with COVID patients and other sick people.
- Many primary care practices, low-cost and free health clinics had been forced to close due to the stress of the pandemic [8, 9].
- 50 million workers were laid off or furloughed, many losing their incomes and health insurance.
- Hospitals had postponed many elective treatments and procedures in order to deal with the influx of COVID patients, resulting in drops in revenue that threatened the survival of safety net hospitals in underserved and rural areas.
- In order to increase the number of hospital beds for COVID patients, some states had closed many psychiatric beds, exacerbating already stressed mental health care.
- Racial inequities had been demonstrated once again, with Black and Hispanic Americans dying of COVID-19 at more than twice the rates of White Americans, as well as experiencing greater economic stress.
- More than 2,900 health care workers had died of COVID-19 [10], while the average life expectancy had declined by a full year [11].
- Job losses in the U.S. were the worst since 1939, with the economy shedding almost 10 million jobs, about twice the losses in 2009 [12].

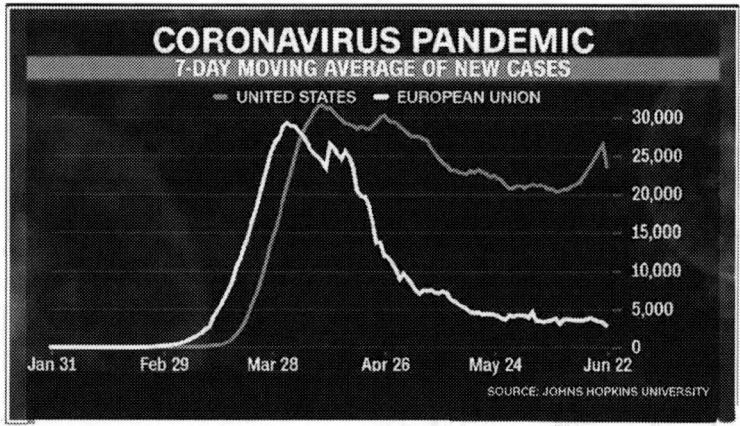

Source: Dr. Sanjay Gupta, *CNN News*, July 27, 2020.

Figure 8.1. Flattening the curve? No way in the USA.

While all that was going on during the first year of the pandemic, profiteering by corporate stakeholders in our medical-industrial complex were putting their self-interest above the public interest, as shown by these examples:

- As the pandemic spread across the country, HCA Healthcare, which owned more than one-half of the most expensive U.S. hospitals, jacked up their charges by as much as 18 times their costs [13].
- Some big pharmaceutical companies saw sharp gains in their stock prices, some more than doubling, through misinformation in their press releases about potential COVID treatments not based on scientific evidence [14].
- Although private insurers were receiving federal payments for COVID testing, critical to control of the pandemic, many insurers profiteered by reimbursing physicians for less than one-half of their costs [15].
- Since many patients were avoiding clinics and hospitals during the pandemic and many elective surgeries were being postponed, large insurers were profiting as never before—the net income for Anthem, as one example, soared to $2.3 billion for the second quarter of 2020, up from $1.1 billion in 2019 [16].

- After Medicare loosened telehealth restrictions early in the pandemic, the program was bilked by billions of dollars in fraudulent claims, according to the U.S. Department of Justice [17].
- Six months into the pandemic, during which almost 1.5 million Americans had suffered with COVID, almost 90,000 dying of it, and 50 million had lost their jobs, billionaire wealth had surged by $845 billion [18].

2.3. Two Years into the Pandemic

- The U.S. was approaching 1 million deaths from COVID out of almost 80 million confirmed cases, with a death rate of 282.8 per 100,000 people (almost three times that of Canada and ten times that of Norway) [19]. Figure 8.2 shows how poorly the U.S. has done in the decline of life expectancy from COVID compared to other countries—36th out of 37 nations [20].

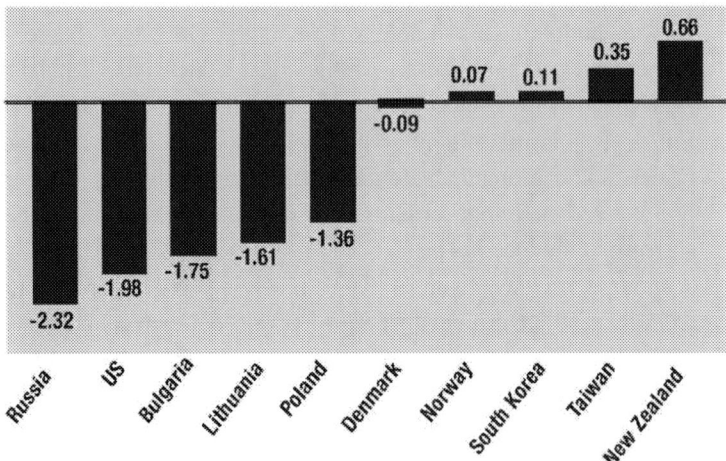

Source: *BMJ* 2021; 375:e066769.

Figure 8.2. Life expectancy fall from COVID-19: Greater in the U.S. than anyplace but Russia.

Poor System Performance during the COVID Pandemic

- COVID death rates varied greatly by state, reflecting marked differences from one state to another in access to care and attitudes about mask-mandates, vaccination, and other preventive approaches [21] (Figure 8.3).

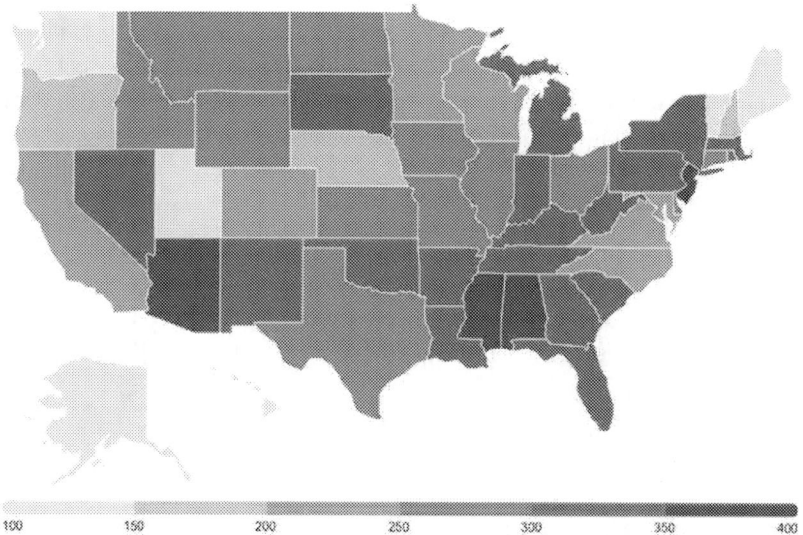

Total COVID-19 deaths per 100,000 people, through Feb. 16, 2022.

Source: Jacobson, L. Charts paint a grim picture 2 years into the coronavirus pandemic. *Kaiser Health News,* March 7, 2022, p. 12.

Figure 8.3. State-by-state death toll from COVID, adjusted for population.

- COVID death rates over a three-month period in early 2022 were more than twice as high in counties where Trump won in a landslide than those where Biden won in a landslide [22].
- Compared to the worldwide average of 56 percent fully vaccinated, 65 percent of Americans were fully vaccinated against COVID by the end of February, 2022 [23]. At this writing, only about one-half of those vaccinated have been boosted [24], and many people, especially in red states, continue to resist vaccination as they assert their "freedom" [25].
- With the omicron subvariant BA.2 spreading rapidly across the country, January of 2022 saw COVID hospitalizations hitting a new

record high at 145,982, and filling about 30% of all ICU beds [26]; at the same time, COVID deaths had topped 2,100 a day [27].
- More than 4,700 health care workers have died after being infected with COVID; understaffing and weakening of safety standards have occurred in many for-profit facilities [28].
- Racial inequities and disparities have persisted throughout the pandemic, as clearly shown by Figure 8.4 [29].
- And, of course, profiteering and even fraud continued to exploit the common good and the public purse, as coronavirus testing scams have left Americans with invalid test results, wrongful medical bills and overpriced at-home tests [30].

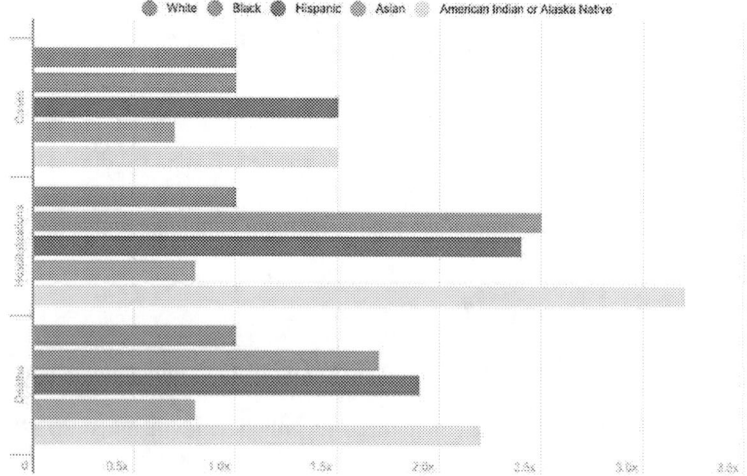

Blacks, Latinos and Native Americans mostly had higher rates of cases, hospitalizations and deaths from COVID-19 than whites did. Asian Americans fared slightly better than whites. Chart shows racial disparities in rates.

Source: Centers for Disease Control and Prevention.

Figure 8.4. People of color in the U.S. were generally hit harder by the pandemic.

3. Some Takeaway Lessons That Can Help Deal with Other Future Pandemics

These are some major points that should underpin serious consideration for reforming U.S. health care.

- *Need to rebuild public health.* Its budget and capabilities have been gutted for many years under both parties. Its present budget of just 3 percent of national health spending should be doubled to 6 percent as an initial way to rebuild its capacity.
- *Need to come together* as a people in a more united way to reduce the differences in response to this and future pandemics. We have to recognize that the virus knows no borders and that we are all in this together.
- *Address systemic racism* —After some 400 years, the importance of this is still made apparent by Figure 8.4 above.
- *Science vs. disinformation*—the rampant misinformation about COVID, its prevention and treatment, needs to be called to account more effectively.
- *Rebuild primary care*—a long-standing challenge that so far has not received enough attention or the national policy priority that it deserves.
- *Rein in profiteering that exploits the public interest*—didn't Chapter 4 make that an urgent priority?
- *Financing reform for universal coverage*, especially important since experience with this pandemic showed that gaps in coverage led to higher numbers of COVID-19 cases, hospitalizations and deaths [31].

Conclusion

The U.S. was clearly ill prepared for the COVID pandemic, which is still with us despite much of public sentiment that has moved on past it. But it is not over, and we are still poorly prepared for the next pandemic, which will come—just a matter of time. COVID has exposed the frailty of our fragmented, dysfunctonal system, our under-developed primary care, our lack of unity in responding to a national emergency, and counter-productive corporate profiteering exploiting the public interest.

Fundamental reform of our health care system is clearly needed, including financing reform that can bring universal coverage. That leads us to the next chapter, but these words from the Editorial Board of *Financial Times*, written more than a year ago when just one year into this pandemic, reminds us of the scope and stakes involved if we are to succeed [32].

> *Beyond defeating the disease the great test that all countries will soon face is whether current feelings of common purpose will shape society after the crisis. As western leaders learnt in the Great Depression, and after the second world war, to demand collective sacrifice you must offer a social contract that benefits everyone.*
>
> *Radical reforms—reversing the prevailing policy direction of the last 4 decades—will need to be put on the table. Governments will have to accept a more active role in the economy. They must see public services as investments rather than liabilities, and look for ways to make labor markets less insecure. Redistribution will again be on the agenda; the privileges of the elderly and wealthy in question. Policies until recently considered eccentric, such as basic income and wealth taxes, will have to be in the mix.*
>
> —Editorial Board of *Financial Times*, April 3, 2020.

References

[1] Press release. Six takeaways of the KHN-AP investigation into the erosion of public health. *Kaiser Health News/Associated Press*, July 1, 2020.

[2] Oberlander, J.As cited by Rovner, J. HealthBent. Always the bridesmaid, public health rarely spotlighted until it's too late. *Kaiser Health News*, May 4, 2020.

[3] Higgins, E. As world joins forces to raise $8 billion for global COVID-19 fund, U.S. contributes this much: $0. *Common Dreams*, May 4, 2020.

[4] Kushner, J. As quoted by Remnick, D. The talk of the town. *The New Yorker*, May 25, 2020, p. 8.

[5] Blumenthal, D. as quoted by Levey, N. Not just the virus: U.S. fails at public health. *Los Angeles Times,* July 6, 2020.

[6] Altman, D. Coronavirus' unequal economic toll. *Axios*, May 29, 2020.

[7] Davidson, K. Deficit reaches $3 trillion as virus costs soar. *Wall Street Journal*, July 14, 2020: A 1.

[8] Ungar, L. Thousands of doctors' offices buckle under the financial stress of COVID. *Kaiser Health News*, November 30, 2020.

[9] Armour, S. Health clinics shut in needy areas. *Wall Street Journal*, July 13, 2020: A 3.

[10] Jewett, C, Lew, R. More than 2,900 health care workers died this year—and the government barely kept track. *Kaiser Health News*, December 23, 2020.

[11] Wamsley, L. American life expectancy dropped by a full year in the first half of 2020. *NPR*, February 18, 2021.

[12] Cambon, SC, Dougherty, D. Job losses in 2020 worst since 1939. *Wall Street Journal*, January 9-10, 2021.

[13] Study finds hospitals hike their charges by up to 18 times costs. *Corporate Crime Reporter* 34 (45): p. 6, November 23, 2020.
[14] Whitfill, T. Biopharma companies are spreading misinformation—and taking advantage of it. *STAT*, May 26, 2020.
[15] Potter, W. Coronavirus pandemic reveals just how devastating the greed of for-profit insurance industry has become. *Common Dreams*, March 18, 2020.
[16] Abelson, R. Major U.S. health insurers report big profits, benefiting from the pandemic. *New York Times*, August 5, 2020.
[17] Eaton, J. Medicare scammers. *AARP Bulletin*, April 2022, p. 22.
[18] Stancil, K. 'Completely upside down': As most Americans struggled during the first six months of the pandemic, billionaire wealth surged by $845 billion. *Common Dreams*, September 17, 2020.
[19] Jacobson, L. Charts paint a grim picture 2 years into the coronavirus pandemic. *Kaiser Health News*, March 7, 2022, p. 12.
[20] Islam, N et al. U.S. ranks 36th out of 37 nations on COVID-19 mortality. *Brit Med J*, 375, 2021.
[21] Ibid # 19, p. 4.
[22] Leonhardt, D. Differences in red and blue America don't hold true in COVID caseloads. *New York Times*, March 10, 2022: A 20.
[23] Visual and data journalism team. COVID map: Coronavirus cases, deaths, vaccinations by country. *BBC News*, February 28, 2022, p. 14.
[24] Schreiber, M. Vastly unequal U.S. has world's highest COVID death toll—it's no coincidence. *The Guardian*, February 6, 2022.
[25] Kates, J, Tolbert, J, Rouw, A. The red/blue divide in COVID-19 vaccination rates continues: An update. *Kaiser Family Foundation*, January 19, 2022.
[26] Stone, W, Feibel, C. U.S. COVID hospitalizations hit new record high, raising risks for patients. *NPR*, January 11, 2022.
[27] Kamp, J. COVID-19 deaths in the U.S. top 2,100 a day, highest in nearly a year. *Wall Street Journal*, January 25, 2022.
[28] Nursing unions say for-profit health care is driving omicron staffing crisis *Truthout*, January 18, 2022.
[29] Ibid # 19, p. 4.
[30] Holpuch, A. Scammers see an opportunity in the demand for coronavirus testing in the U.S., officials say. *New York Times*, January 16, 2022.
[31] Campbell, Travis and P. Galvani, Alison and Fitzpatrick, Meagan and Friedman, Gerald. The role of the fragmented United States healthcare system in exacerbating COVID-19 mortality. *Lancet*. January 5, 2022.
[32] Editorial Board. Virus lays bare the frailty of the social contract. Radical reforms are required to forge a society that will work for all. *Financial Times*, April 3, 2020: 150.

Chapter 9

Failed Multi-Payer Financing Systems for U.S. Health Care

> *Illness is an unpredictable risk for the individual family, but we know fairly accurately how much illness a large group of people will have, how much medical care they will require, and how many days they will have to spend in hospitals. In other words, we cannot budget the cost of illness per individual family but we can budget it for the nation. The principle must be to spread the risk among as many people as possible . . . The experience of the last 15 years in the United States [since 1931] has, in my opinion, demonstrated that voluntary health insurance does not solve the problem of the nation. It reaches only certain groups and is always at the mercy of economic fluctuations . . . Hence, if we decide to finance medical services through insurance, the insurance system must be compulsory.*
>
> —Dr. Henry Sigerist, as Director of the History of Medicine at the Johns Hopkins University in 1944 [1]

As the costs of medical care and health insurance have skyrocketed over the last two decades in this country, the largely private health insurance industry has come under scrutiny as a major part of the problem. This chapter has just two goals: (1) to give some historical background to the development of private health insurance within our multi-payer financing system; and (2) to show how the multi-payer financing system has failed the public interest.

1. Brief Historical Background

The above opening quote by Dr. Sigerist in the mid-1940s highlights a key issue—the need for the widest possible sharing of risk through compulsory health insurance. Three decades earlier, 10 European countries had adopted one or another form of compulsory health insurance. A progressive movement before World War I in the U.S. favored that approach, but it was soon dropped as the war took center stage. Fast forward to today, and the U.S. has still not effectively addressed the question of compulsory vs. voluntary. Instead, an enormous largely private health insurance industry has evolved with enough political power and lobbyists to continue sidelining the issue.

Health insurance started in the U.S. during the Great Depression with the emergence of a not-for-profit Blue Cross plan for school teachers in Dallas, Texas in 1929. That so-called voluntary Baylor plan provided free hospitalization for up to 21 days at a time, with the hospital assuming financial risk. Other pre-paid insurance plans came along during the 1930s, when the nation's hospitals were in dire straits with more than one-third of their general hospital beds empty [2]. The World War II years saw the emergence of employer-sponsored health insurance when employers found it helpful to provide health insurance to recruit workers during the severe labor shortage of the wartime economy.

From the beginning, most economists have adopted the conventional theory of insurance, based on moral hazard, which holds that people with insurance will overuse health care services. The concept of "consumer directed health care" has therefore become widely adopted, with the assumption that such overuse can be controlled by cost sharing whereby enrollees have enough "skin in the game" [3].

Although early health insurers tended to be not-for-profit and supportive of guaranteed coverage and community rating, that approach was replaced during and after the 1960s with the widespread use of medical underwriting in order to avoid covering higher risk individuals. The flood gates were thereby opened as insurers put profits before service, gained investors on Wall Street, and used increased cost sharing at the point of service through deductibles and co-payments.

Medicare and Medicaid were enacted in 1965 as important public programs, but were later targets for privatization by insurers whereby enrollees' choice and coverage were reduced in order to increase insurers' revenues. The 1990s saw another major opportunity to expand their reach and revenues through managed care with the development of health maintenance organizations (HMOs). They were intended to contain health care costs by changing from fee-for-service payment to prospective payment based on capitation—the number of individuals enrolled in each HMO [4]. That supposed attempt for cost containment, however, soon fell victim to quite the opposite—continued exploitation of public programs at taxpayer expense.

The industry grew to as many as 1,300 private health insurers at one point, but has decreased to smaller numbers of ever-larger companies through consolidation. In so doing, the risk pool is fragmented into smaller and smaller parts as insurers work to avoid adverse selection in order to increase their profits. Consolidation also can bring with it broadened reach into other health care sectors, with increased market power to set prices. As one example, Anthem, which owns Blue Cross Blue Shield in 14 states as well as IngenioRx, a drug benefit manager, recently acquired Beacon HealthOptions, a behavioral health company and myNEXUS, which manages home-based health care [5].

2. How Multi-Payer Financing Has Failed the Public Interest

As a result, we now have a largely private for-profit health insurance industry at increasingly unaffordable and unsustainable costs to patients, families and taxpayers. The largest single part of it has been employer-sponsored insurance, which has been subsidized by the federal government for many years, currently at about $685 billion a year [6], a number that is projected by the Congressional Budget Office to double in another 10 years [7].

These are some of the major ways by which private health insurers and multi-payer financing of health care have failed the common good in this country.

2.1. Unaffordable Costs

The costs of health insurance have become increasingly unaffordable for years, having gone up much faster than wages for many years, as shown by Figure 9.1 since 2000. In 2018, they grew by 15 percent in just one year [8]. In 2019, the average family of four with employer-sponsored health insurance through a preferred provider organization (PPO) was paying an average of $28,653 a year for health care, including insurance premiums, cost sharing and forgone wage increases for the employer contribution. That was a heavy burden since the median household income at that time was $66,500 [9]. In 2020, the average premium alone paid by the employer and employee for a family plan topped $20,000, with the enrollee contributing about $5,500 [10]. As a result of these high costs, four in ten people with employer-sponsored insurance don't have enough savings to cover the deductibles, while one in six have to cut back on food, take an extra job, or move in with friends or family [11].

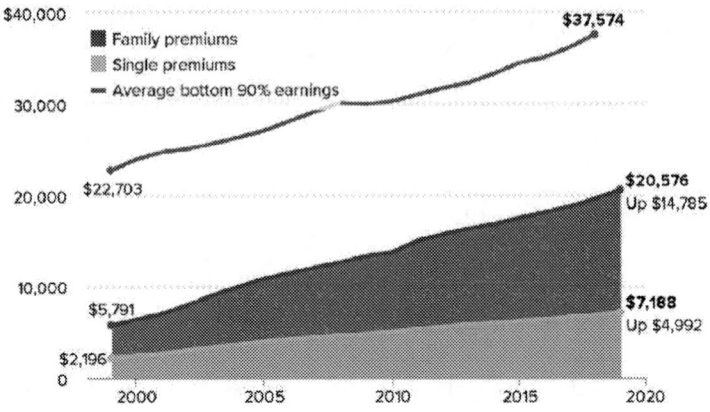

Source: Kaiser Family Foundation.

Figure 9.1. Workers' health insurance premiums are rising much faster than wages.

2.2. Growth of a Denial Industry

Even when insured, enrollees cannot have confidence in having coverage when they need it. Insurers have developed many ways to deny physicians' and hospitals' claims for services already provided. They increasingly require pre-authorization of services before they can be paid, often based on ever-changing networks about which physicians and patients are often one step behind. Out-of-networks claims are often unaffordable; even for in-network claims, the average denial rate is now 18 percent [12].

2.3. Privatization of Public Programs

Medicare and Medicaid have been raided by private insurers for more than three decades based on the false premise that they can be more efficient than their public counterparts. That has led, in every instance, to restricted choice and coverage, volatility of coverage, and administrative overhead five to six times higher than for traditional Medicare. In their quest for profits, they have often "up-coded" diagnoses in order to claim payment for conditions for which care was not provided. See Table 4.1 for how this scam works [13]. Recall from Figure 2.2 in Chapter 2 how our 5 largest insurers were being kept afloat at taxpayer expense from 2010 to 2016 [14].

2.4. Inadequate Benefits

Despite their high costs, private health insurers fall far short of offering comprehensive benefits, as these examples illustrate:

- Benefits under employer-sponsored insurance keep diminishing as employers limit benefits and as employees pay more in lost wages.
- Even when insurers claim to cover prescription drugs, a recent national poll found that they deny covering prescriptions for more than one-third of adults across all income groups [15].
- Women's health care coverage is often limited in both private and Medicaid plans, so that women frequently skip needed care—a major factor in U.S. women having a very high maternal mortality rate (# 46 in the world) [16].
- Mental health coverage is often lacking as insurers keep very minimal lists of in-network providers, typically forcing patients to pay large out-of-pocket costs to out-of-network providers [17].
- Long-term care coverage is usually uncovered, as is also the case for Medicare; Medicaid covers more of its costs, but only after patients have spent down to poverty level.
- Short-term plans: these are designed to get around requirements of the Affordable Care Act and are correctly labeled as "junk insurance," offering very limited coverage at exorbitant costs for up to one year. Under the deceptive name of Golden Rule Insurance, they have been very profitable to its owner, UnitedHealth Group [18].

2.5. Profiteering, Even Fraud

Overall, private health insurers consume 15 to 20 percent of the health care dollar in bureaucracy, administrative overhead and profits. They have many ways to profiteer, including when not actually providing coverage.

Gerald Friedman, Professor of Economics at the University of Massachusetts Amherst and author of *The Case for Medicare for All*, notes the way they do that:

> *Rather than increasing sales, health insurers profit by screening customers, segmenting the market so as to exclude those likely to use health care ("lemon dropping") while attracting the healthy and lucky who use less health care ("cherry picking")* [19].

Private insurers accomplish the "cherry picking" goal through restrictive underwriting, narrow networks, denial of coverage and services, deceptive marketing practices, and bloated administrative costs. Figure 6.5 shows how much higher their administrative overhead is compared to five other countries.

Privatized Medicare and Medicaid have been a bonanza for private insurers for many years. Insurers have partnered with third-party vendors to perform medical chart reviews to find thousands of extra diagnostic codes that can be claimed for overpayments [20]. They have also successfully lobbied Congress for ever-higher overpayments, in part based upon fraudulent up-coding of diagnoses and claiming payment for conditions for which treatment was not given. These overpayments have become built into the "system" to the point that they surged after passage of the Affordable Care Act in 2010 [21]. Overpayments to private Medicaid managed care plans are endemic in more than 30 states, usually involving unnecessary or duplicative payments to providers [22].

Remarkably and inappropriately, United Health, one of the largest of U.S. private health insurers, has been working to Americanize the U.K.'s National Health Service (NHS) for the last 10 years through its Global Health Division. It is promoting new care models there—essentially rebranded HMO—attempting to convert the NHS to a publicly funded, privately controlled and delivered corporate cash cow resembling Medicare Advantage and Medicaid Managed Care in this country [23].

2.6. Unreliability and Volatility

In their quest for increased revenues, corporate private health insurers are prone to leave their markets, often with little advance notice, when their profits fall below expectations of their CEOs and shareholders. As one example, at least 1.4 million people in 32 states lost their coverage under the Affordable

Care Act at the end of 2016, leaving them with fewer choices than before [24]. Private Medicare Advantage plans are another example of unreliability. After cherry-picking enrollees in the first place, they often disenroll them when they become sicker and less profitable [25].

Employer-sponsored health insurance, though still the largest part of the industry, is unstable and on a decline for many reasons, including the volatility of workers' employment—by age 50, they have held an average of 12 jobs—and the instability of the economy, more so during this COVID pandemic, with many lost jobs likely to be gone for good [26]. That has led to Dr. Atul Gawande, surgeon, public health researcher, and author of *Being Mortal: Medicine and What Matters in the End*, to this astute observation:

> *The central error of our system has been attaching our health care to where we work. A company-sponsored insurance plan for a family adds an average of fifteen thousand dollars to the annual cost of employing a worker—effectively levying a fifty-per-cent tax on a fifteen-dollar-an-hour position. We're all but paying employers to outsource or automate people's jobs. The result is to make both work and health care less secure and more fragmented—and to deepen our inequalities* [27].

Table 9.1 lists reasons that private health insurance does not meet the needs of coverage for all Americans and should be considered obsolete [28], as will be further discussed in Chapter 13.

Table 9.1. Why private health insurance is obsolete

- Inefficiencies vs public-financing
- Fragments risk pools by medical underwriting
- Increasing epidemic of underinsurance
- Excessive administrative and overhead costs
- Profiteering—shareholders trump patients
- Pricing itself out of the market
- Unsustainable and resists regulation

In summary, these are some of the main reasons that our present financing system is in urgent need for fundamental reform:

- A flawed financing system, with many ways for providers, vendors and corporate stakeholders to game the system for their own self-interest.
- High, unaffordable prices and costs, with cost containment nowhere on the horizon.
- Rationing of care by ability to pay (or non-ability!) to pay.
- Unemployment during the pandemic reminiscent of Great Depression levels of the 1930s.
- 87 million Americans already underinsured before the pandemic.
- Serious shortages in primary care and psychiatry, partly due to under-reimbursement, with no national physician workforce plan yet in place to meet system needs.
- Many stressed hospitals closing, especially in rural and underserved areas.

Conclusion

The corporate transformation of U.S. health care over the last 60 years has brought us increased urgency for fundamental system reform. We can expect that all efforts in this direction will be hard fought by corporate stakeholders, their Wall Street handlers, and well-funded lobbyists. We will see in the next chapter just how those forces pursue their self-interest at the expense of the common good.

References

[1] Sigerist, H. Medical care for all the people. *Canadian Journal of Public Health* 35 (7): 258, 1944.
[2] Stuart, JE. *The Blue Cross Story: An Informal Biography of the Voluntary Prepayment Plan for Hospital Care*. Chicago. BCBSA Archives. Photocopied typescript, circa 1966, p. 19.
[3] Geyman, JP. Moral hazard and consumer-driven health care: A fundamentally flawed concept. *Intl J Health Services* 37 (2): 333-351, 2007.

[4] Jensen, Gail A, Michael A Morrisey, Shannon Gaffney, and Derek K Liston. The new dominance of managed care: Insurance trends in the 1990s. *Health Affairs (Millwood)* 16 (1): 135-136, 1997.
[5] Mathews, AW. Anthem looks to diversify, rename itself Elevance Health. *Wall Street Journal*, March 11, 2022: B 2.
[6] Ockerman, E. It costs $685 billion a year to subsidize U.S. health insurance. *Bloomberg News*, May 23, 2018.
[7] Potter, W. Take it from me, tweaks won't fix health care. *USA Today*, December 14, 2018.
[8] Bruenig, M. People lose their employer-sponsored insurance constantly. *People's Policy Project*, April 4, 2019.
[9] Girod, CS, Hart, SK, Liner, DM. 2019 Milliman Medical Index. *Milliman Research Report*. December 2019.
[10] Mathews, AW. Health coverage costs are rising. *Wall Street Journal*, October 9, 2020: A 2.
[11] Levey, NN. Health insurance deductibles soar, leaving Americans with unaffordable bills. *Los Angeles Times*, May 2, 2019.
[12] Silvers, JB. This is the most realistic path to Medicare for All. *New York Times*, October 16, 2019.
[13] Schulte, F, Donald, D. Cracking the codes: How doctors and hospitals have collected billions in questionable Medicare fees. *Center for Public Integrity*, May 19, 2014.
[14] Schoen, C, Collins, SR. The Big Five health insurers' membership and revenue trends: Implications for public policy. *Health Affairs* 36 (2), December, 2017.
[15] Neighmond, P. When insurance won't cover drugs, Americans make 'tough choices' about their health. *NPR*, January 27, 2020.
[16] Gunja, Munira Z, Shanoor Seervai, Laurie Zephyrin, Reginald D Williams II. Issue Brief. Health and health care for women of reproductive age: How the United States compares with other high-income countries. New York. *The Commonwealth Fund*, April 6, 2022.
[17] Boyd, JW. Having health insurance doesn't mean mental health care access. Chicago, IL. Physicians for a National Health Program. *PNHP Newsletter*, Fall 2019, pp. 20-21.
[18] Hiltzik, M. Why short-term health plans are cheap: They shortchange you on care. *Los Angeles Times*, August 12, 2019.
[19] Friedman, G. An open letter to the *New York Times* that was rejected. February 6, 2016.
[20] Schulte, F, Weber, L. Medicare Advantage overbills taxpayers by billions a year as feds struggle to stop it. *Kaiser Health News*, July 16, 2019.
[21] Geruso, M, Layton, T. Upcoding inflates Medicare costs in excess of $2 billion annually. *UT News*, University of Texas at Austin, June 18, 2015.
[22] Herman, B. Medicaid's unmanaged managed care. *Modern Healthcare*, April 30, 2016.
[23] Player, S, Gill, B. U.S. empire seized U.K.'s National Health Service. *Consortium News* 26 (354), December 11, 2021.

[24] Tracer, Z, Darie, T. More than 1 million in Obamacare lose plans as insurers quit. *Bloomberg News*, October 14, 2016.
[25] Schulte, F. As seniors get sicker, they're more likely to drop Medicare Advantage plans. *Kaiser Health News*, July 6, 2017.
[26] Cohen, P. Many jobs may vanish forever as layoffs mount. *New York Times*, May 21, 2020.
[27] Gawande, A. A Nation's Health Care: Rescuing the System. *The New Yorker*, October 5, 2020, pp. 12-13.
[28] Geyman, JP. *Do Not Resuscitate: Why the Health Insurance Industry Is Dying, and How We Must Replace It*. Monroe, ME. *Common Courage Press*, 2008, p. 112.

Chapter 10

How Wall Street and Corporate Interests Extract Profits and Professionalism from Health Care

As you recall, we took a quick tour across the medical-industrial complex of privatization, profiteering, corruption and fraud in Chapter 4. Here we will focus on investor-owned health care as taken over by Wall Street-based private equity to the detriment of patients, families, physicians and other health care professionals. This chapter has three goals: (1) to bring historical perspective to transformative changes in U.S. health care that have followed the intrusion of Wall Street-based corporate stakeholders into the delivery of health care services; (2) to describe private equity, the worst of the Wall Street-based villains, as it harms patient care with its unbounded corporate greed; and (3) to consider how this new profit-driven clinical environment has distorted the doctor-patient relationship and medical practice itself.

1. Some Historical Perspective

These observations at intervals over more than 40 plus years bring a useful overview to the transformative changes of U.S. health care that have occurred in that time period.

1980:

> *By the end of the 1980s, Wall Street had permanently changed corporate America. A new type of business model existed. The leveraged buyout industry, stung with bad publicity, rebranded as "private equity." While some PE firms made productive investments, they were largely tools of floating capital that sought to use the corporation for the purpose of financier* [1].

> —Matt Stoller, former senior policy advisor and budget analyst to the Senate Budget Committee and author of *Goliath: The 100-Year War between Monopoly Power and Democracy*

1999:

Consider what has happened to American medicine over the past thirty years. The physician's relationship to patients has been drastically altered. Medicine's traditional methods of controlling economic competition and making a living have been largely been destroyed. Independent, solo, fee-for-service practice is rapidly disappearing. The clinical freedom of the physician has been seriously weakened. Divisions within the profession have intensified. Taken together, these changes have the potential to destroy professionalism in medicine and reduce physicians to the position of technicians [2].

—the late Eliot Friedson, PhD, Professor Emeritus of Sociology, New York University, and author of *Profession of Medicine: A Study of the Sociology of Applied Knowledge*

Perhaps the most extraordinary development in medical practice during the age of managed care was that time, in the name of efficiency, was being squeezed out of the doctor-patient relationship. Managed care organizations, with their insistence on maximizing "throughput," were forcing physicians to churn through patients in assembly-line fashion at ever-accelerating rates of speed. . . In 1997, doctors on average spent eight minutes talking to each patient, less than half as much time as a decade before [3].

—Kenneth Ludmerer, M.D., internist, medical historian, and Professor of Medicine at Washington University in St. Louis

In the profit-maximizing milieu of American medicine, capitation risks make things even worse. "Risk-sharing" too often means that physicians earn bonuses for denying care—a danger perceived by patients, who take a dim view of capitation. Risk-sharing is not simply the inverse of fee-for-service, but of fee-splitting, the illegal practice of kickbacks for referrals.

—Drs. David Himmelstein and Steffie Woolhandler, general internists, health policy experts, and co-founders of Physicians for a National Health Program [4]

> *During the 1990s, the delivery of health care services was increasingly influenced by the demands of investors and investor-owned firms. A growing number of hospitals, health maintenance organizations (HMOs), nursing homes, home care services, and hospices became for-profit companies, publicly traded on stock exchanges. Companies formed to fill niches, such as those that manage physicians' practices and utilization review firms, became Wall Street favorites. The buying and selling of health-industry assets, as fungible commodities, intensified. In the meantime, traditional for-profit entities such as medical device and drug companies continued to thrive. In the early part of the decade, the performance of health care stocks exceeded that of the market as a whole* [5].
>
> —Robert Kuttner, leading economist, founder and co-editor of *The American Prospect*, and author of the 2007 book, *Everything for Sale and the End of Laissez-Faire*

2007:

> *Health care in America is in deep crisis. A public service has been transformed into a for-profit enterprise in which physicians are "health care providers," patients are consumers, and both subserve corporate interests. The effect has been to convert medicine into a business, de-professionalize doctors and far worse, depersonalize patients* [6].
>
> —Bernard Lown, M.D., cardiologist, developer of the cardiac defibrillator, and recipient of the Nobel Peace Prize in 1985

2. How Private Equity Harms Patient Care for Short-Term Investors' Gain

In recent decades, Wall Street corporate interests have taken advantage of our deregulated market-based system to steal professionalism out of health care and amass profits for investors through private equity. That process has metastasized across our system ranging from hospitals and nursing homes to emergency care, mental health, home care and elsewhere. In so doing, the constant result is higher prices and costs, lower quality of care, planned instability, and further fragmentation of health care. Jim Hightower, author of *The Hightower Lowdown*, describes their typical operations this way:

> *With some notable exceptions, the business of hedge funds and private equity outfits is corporate plunder: They amass a pile of money from big investors and banks and use it to buy foundering businesses on the cheap; slash workforces; degrade quality; jack up prices . . .* [7]

An in-depth working paper from the Center for Economic and Policy Research in 2020 gave us a birds' eye view of the scope and damages of private equity buyouts in this country. It described these four main segments where private equity has been especially active:

1. Hospitals;
2. Outpatient care (urgent care and ambulatory surgery centers);
3. Physician staffing and emergency room services (surprise medical billing); and
4. Revenue cycle management (medical debt collecting).

In each of these segments, we are told that:

> *Private equity has taken the lead in consolidating small providers, loading them with debt, and rolling them up into large powerhouses with substantial market power before exiting with handsome returns* [8].

Health care was the second major sector for private equity investment in 2020, accounting for 18 percent of all reported deals. From 2010 to 2020, the number of these deals increased by more than 250 percent (Figure 10.1) [9]. Figure 10.2 shows the comparative amounts of capital invested by segment between 2000 and 2019 [10].

In the last 10 years, private equity investments have been a leading force in mergers, acquisitions and the consolidation of physicians as providers in an effort to gain market power in local, regional and national markets. Since 2013, private equity investments have shifted from hospitals to clinics and outpatient services. "Other healthcare services" includes small physician specialty practices, which now accounts for about 40 percent of all investments in this period [11].

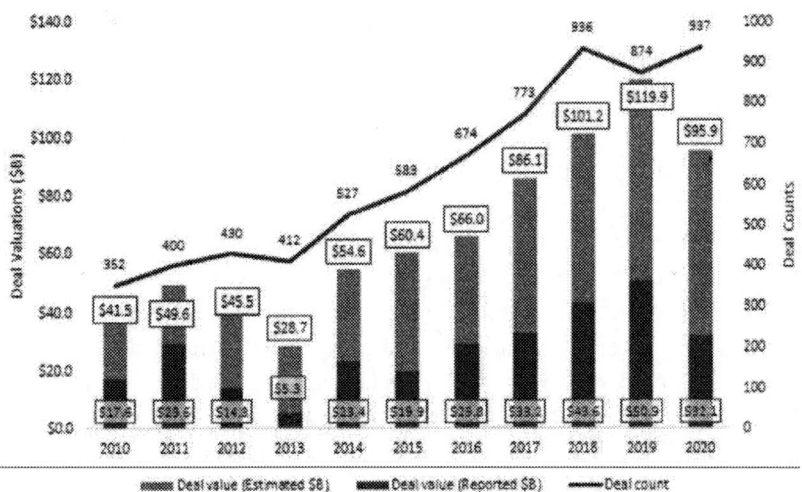

Figure 10.1. Total PE deals in healthcare: reported deal value, estimated deal value, and reported deal count, 2010-2020.

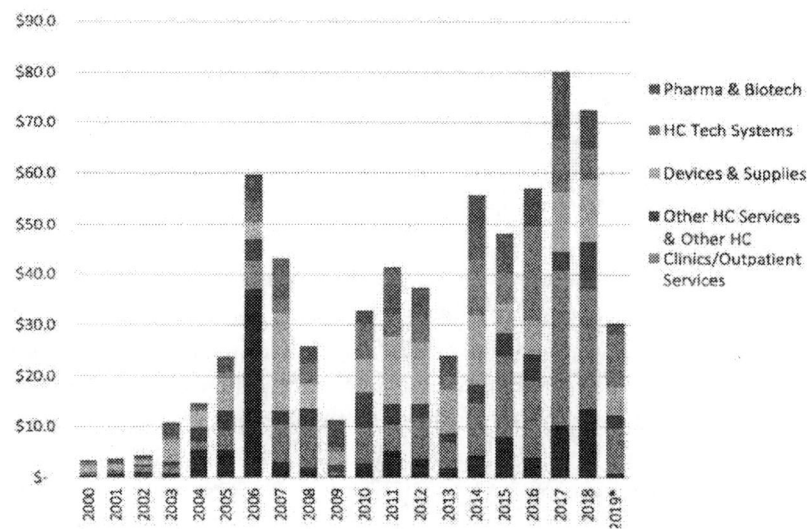

*Source: PitqhBook data, as of October, W19.
Source: Appelbaum, E, Batt, R. "Private equity buyouts in healthcare: Who wins, who loses". *Working Paper No. 118, Center for Economic and Policy Research and Institute for New Economic Thinking*, March 15, 2020.

Figure 10.2. Private equity capital invested by segment: 2000-2019.

Here are examples of the nefarious takeovers of physician practices by private equity firms that end badly for the involved physicians:

- Envision Healthcare, the largest U.S. physician staffing firm, specializes in emergency department staffing through its subsidiary EmCare. After its takeovers, emergency room physicians are "outsourced" in not being part of any insurer's network. As a result, EmCare has been able to send very high surprise out-of-network bills even when their hospitals were in the insurer's network. A study by Yale University researchers found that those pricing practices led to an 83 percent increase in patient cost sharing after EmCare contracted with hospitals [12]. That led to increasing scrutiny, loss of creditors, a bill introduced in Congress to end surprise medical bills, worries of bankruptcy, lawsuit in California December 2021, and understaffing of ERs with potential deadly impacts on patients [13].
- Buying dermatology [14], obstetrics-gynecology [15], and ophthalmology [16] practices, holding them for three to seven years, during which physicians are pressured to see more patients and do more procedures in order to extract maximal profits while gaining more negotiating power with insurers, then selling the practices for higher prices.
- Other specialties impacted by private equity involvement in mergers and acquisitions include anesthesiology, dentistry, gastroenterology, orthopedic surgery, and radiology [17].

Nursing homes, home health care and hospice companies have recently become priority for private equity investments, largely because of their reliable sources of revenue (mostly Medicare) and profit potential. In the home healthcare industry, private equity was involved in almost one-half of deals between 2018 and 2019. Under private equity ownership, staffing is typically cut, workers are paid less, and quality of patient care suffers. Hospitalizations increase from nursing homes while the number of visits are reduced during patients' final days in hospice. Their owners and executives are often bought off by "dividend recapitalization," whereby they are paid well in dividends by taking on new debt [18].

Primary care is another recent target for private equity investment with the promised goal to "save money while improving patient care." The current federal "value-based" payment system being used by Medicare is based on criteria for patients' improvement, not the number of services provided, again in hopes of saving money. VillageMD, focused on the management of chronic disease, is one such venture-backed company toward that goal, now serving 1.6 million patients in more than 250 locations. Annie Lamont, co-founder of another venture-backed firm, Oak HC/FT, adds to its goal: "It really is about moving the center of gravity from patients being managed by hospital systems to really being managed by primary care doctors" [19].

CVS Health, parent of insurer Aetna, plans to put primary care physicians in 350 of its retail stores. United Health's Optum unit has more than 60,000 employed or "aligned" physicians, about one-half in primary care [20].

Despite this supposed "progress," however, these developments have not yet been shown to really improve patient care, and can neither be counted upon to provide continuity of comprehensive care nor continuity of any physician-patient relationships. Dr. Zirui Song, a primary care physician at Massachusetts General Hospital and Associate Professor of Health Care Policy at Harvard Medical School, raises this concern:

> *The trust between a patient and a primary care clinician is especially important for the patient's care trajectory through the health care system. If private equity somehow infringes on that relationship of trust between a patient and their health care providers, especially their primary care provider, then society should be more concerned about the current influx of private equity acquisitions within health care* [21].

The private equity industry lacks transparency and accountability largely because it is unregulated under state and federal law. These venture capital companies describe their role as management services organizations (MSO's) that buy up and manage financial assets of acquired holdings but delegate leadership to a chief medical officer whom they hire as partners, but who also can be fired [22].

A 2021 report from the American Antitrust Institute and the Petris Center at the University of California Berkeley cautioned that:

> *The implications of a forecasted increase in private equity investment in healthcare are concerning. The pandemic has weakened many parts of the health system even with financial aid provided by the government, and small physician practices and other less capitalized firms in outpatient care may be under particular strain. Private equity firms such as Audax Group ($15B in dry powder) that specialize in growing outpatient care companies through aggressive acquisition*

strategies may find themselves in a buyer's market as they seek to acquire small physician groups struggling with high overhead costs and pandemic-related debts [23].

3. Adverse Impacts on Physicians, Their Practices and Other Health Professionals

In view of the above trends, the value system in U.S. health care has clearly shifted from a service ethic to unbridled monetary gain, especially for corporate stakeholders and their investors at the expense of continuity and quality of patient care. The value of what used to be a long-lasting doctor-patient relationship has been a casualty of these trends.

According to physician surveys carried out by the AMA, the proportion of U.S. physicians owning their own practices dropped from more than 75 percent in 1983 to 46 percent in 2018. At the start of 2021, 70 percent of U.S. physicians worked for health systems or corporate owners, an increase from about 62 percent in 2019 [24]. That has resulted in fewer places for patients to seek care, with most of those available today in more impersonal mega-facilities. Deborah Goldman, a visiting fellow at the Ethics and Public Policy Center, observes:

> *The replacement of the small doctor's office with large-scale facilities hasn't made medicine cheaper or access to it easier. It threatens to remove a core advantage of the small, privately owned practice: the sense of personal, immediate responsibility between physician and patient* [25].

For physicians, these changes have meant more fragmentation and volatility of care, loss of clinical autonomy, and declining practice satisfaction. As we saw in Chapter 5, they have also led to increased burnout rates and early retirements [26].

Can these adverse impacts be reversed? Unfortunately, not at all likely, given the power of money and the deep pockets of Wall Street interests. They have penetrated to the heart of medicine and health care. The classic traditions of the medical profession have been trampled upon, leaving an open question whether those traditions can be re-established by health care reform. Reform will be difficult to achieve, as we will see in later chapters.

Conclusion

The market theory of health care has exploited and abandoned the public interest. It does not fit the goals, principles and ethics of medicine and health care. It is harmful to patients, physicians and their profession alike. The "system" is a mess, and all previous efforts to effectively reform it have failed. As Dr. Marcia Angell, former editor of *The New England Journal of Medicine* and author of *The Truth about Drug Companies: How They Deceive Us and What We Can Do About It*, said 20 years ago.

> *We've engaged in a massive and failed experiment in market-based medicine in the U.S. Rhetoric about the benefits of competition and profit-driven health care can no longer hide the reality: Our health system is in shambles* [27].

Since that comment two decades ago, the shambles are still here, if not worse. That raises the question whether or not regulation could be effective, which we will try to answer in the next chapter.

References

[1] Stoller, M. *Goliath: The 100-Year War between Monopoly Power and Democracy.* New York. *Simon & Schuster*, 2019, p. 405.
[2] Friedson, EL. Professionalism and institutional ethics. In Baker, RB, Caplan, AL, Emanuel, LL & Latham, SR (eds.). *The American Medical Ethics Revolution.* Baltimore: *Johns Hopkins Press*, 1999: 130-131.
[3] Ludmerer, KM. *Time to Heal: American Medical Education from the Turn of the Century to the Era of Managed Care.* New York. *Oxford University Press*, 1999, p.384.
[4] Himmelstein, DU, Woolhandler, S. Global amnesia: embracing fee-for-non-service—again. *J Gen Intern Med*, January 7, 2014.
[5] Kuttner, R. The American Health Care System: Wall Street and Health Care. *New Engl J Med* 34 (8), 664, 1999.
[6] Lown, B. The commodification of health care. *PNHP Newsletter*, 2007.
[7] Hightower, J. The priority is profit. *The Hightower Lowdown*, January 2020, pp. 1-2.
[8] Appelbaum, E, Batt, R. *Private equity buyouts in healthcare: Who wins, who loses.* Working Paper No. 118, Center for Economic and Policy Research and Institute for New Economic Thinking, March 15, 2020.
[9] Scheffler, RM, Alexander, LM, Godwin, JR. Soaring private equity investment in the healthcare sector: Consolidation accelerated, competition undermined, and

patients at risk. *American Antitrust Institute and Petris Center, School of Public Health, University of California, Berkeley*, May 18, 2021, pp. 8-9.
[10] Ibid #8, 19-21
[11] Ibid # 9, p. 11.
[12] Cooper, Z, Scott Morton, E, Shekita, N. Surprise! Out-of-network billing for emergency care in the United States. *J of Political Economy* 128 (9): 3626-3677, 2020.
[13] Applebaum, E, Batt, R. Envision healthcare hits the skids. *The American Prospect*, March 14, 2022.
[14] Meyer, H. Concerns grow as private equity buys up dermatology practices. *Modern Healthcare*, July 24, 2017.
[15] Bruch, Joseph D, Alexander Borsa, Zirui Song, Sarah S Richardson. Expansion of private equity involvement in women's health care. *JAMA Internal Medicine*, August 24, 2020.
[16] O'Donnell, Eloise May, Gary Joseph Lelli, Sami Bhidya, Lawrence P Casalino. The growth of private equity investment in health care: Perspectives from ophthalmology. *Health Affairs* 39 (6), June, 2020.
[17] Ibid # 8, p. 4.
[18] Johnson, J. Report rings alarm over private equity's grip on home health, hospice industries. *Common Dreams*, March 18, 2022.
[19] Lamont, A. As quoted by Peebles, A. Why investors are pouring billions into primary care. *Bloomberg News*, February 24, 2022.
[20] Peebles, A. Your primary care doctor may soon be working for Wall Street, or at CVS. *Seattle Times*, February 11, 2022.
[21] Song, Z. As quoted by Peebles, A., Ibid # 18.
[22] Ibid # 8, p. 5.
[23] Ibid # 9, p. 11.
[24] Daily Briefing. Why investors are pouring billions into primary care. *Advisory Board.* February 24, 2022.
[25] Goldman, D. The doctor's office becomes an assembly line. *Wall Street Journal*, December 30, 2021: A 17.
[26] Kane, L. *Medscape National Physician Burnout, Depression and Suicide Report*, 2019, January 16, 2019.
[27] Angell, M. Sweeping health care reform proposed by nation's top physicians. Press release. *Physicians for a National Health Program*, Chicago, IL, May 1, 2001.

Chapter 11

Barriers to System Reform

> *It has become difficult not to recognize that we are firmly in the grip of a second Gilded Age. Not only is this return obvious in the homage— if not hysteria—that marks a return to the dream worlds of consumption, commodification and survival-of-the-fittest ethic, but also in the actions of right-wing politicians who want to initiate policies that take the country back to the late 19th century—a time in which the reforms of the New Deal, the Great Society and the Progressive Era did not exist* [1].

—Henry A. Giroux, Professor of English and Cultural Studies at McMaster University, Hamilton, Ontario and author of *Politics after Hope: Obama and the Crisis of Youth, Race and Democracy*

In the broadest overview, as articulated in 2011 by Professor Giroux above, this may help to explain the failure of reform attempts in the past, the actions (or non-actions!) of today's GOP, and the challenges to future reform initiatives in health care. This chapter has three goals: (1) to discuss how health care reform has failed in the past; (2) to consider lessons that we can learn from the failures of those attempts; and (3) to discuss the obstacles facing reform attempts today.

1. How Reform Has Failed in the Past

As you have seen in earlier chapters, the excesses of the "free market" in fueling increasingly unaffordable prices and costs of U.S. health care, together with reduced access and its related problems, have been with us for many decades. That is not to say that there have not been many attempts to bring them under control in a reformed system. In every case, however, organized opposition led to their defeat for reasons that we can learn from today.

The real fix will be enacting a financing system of universal coverage, as other advanced countries discovered long ago. These are the major attempts that go back more than a century to address that goal in this country:

1. In 1912, as a presidential candidate on the progressive ticket, Teddy Roosevelt proposed national health insurance, later taken up by progressives in 1916. Although a committee of the AMA had initially supported national health insurance (NHI) in 1917 [2], growing opposition to it by state chapters around the country led the national organization to strongly oppose it then (and in later years) [3]. Labor sided with business and organized medicine to defeat NHI in 1917, which was also sidelined as national priorities shifted to World War I [4]. Opponents also fear mongered that it was the nation's greatest international threat [5].
2. In the mid-1930s, Franklin Delano Roosevelt proposed NHI, initially attached to Social Security as part of his New Deal legislative package. Confronted by strong opposition to NHI by the AMA, however, FDR decided to go ahead with Social Security without a provision for it [6].
3. In 1944, FDR called for "an economic bill of rights" in his State of the Union message, including a plan for "adequate medical care" for all Americans. After his death in April, 1945, incoming President Harry Truman brought forward a proposed compulsory plan for comprehensive national health insurance. Opponents quickly organized themselves through the leadership of large corporations, the AMA, the American Hospital Association, the American Bar Association, and the Chamber of Commerce. Opponents demonized NHI as socialism, while the AMA went so far as to claim that NHI "would turn physicians into slaves" [7]. All that succeeded in turning the voting public to favor *voluntary* health insurance over the *compulsory* proposal [8].
4. In 1971, Senator Teddy Kennedy introduced a Health Security Act with a single-payer public financing system for universal coverage. It was a competing bill with the AMA's Medicredit proposal and the Kerr-Mills compromise proposal, none of which were passed as the country's attention became focused on Watergate and the Vietnam War [9].
5. During the 1976 presidential elections, Jimmy Carter campaigned for NHI.
6. In 1994, during the Clinton presidency, the McDermott-Conyers-Wellstone single-payer bill for national health insurance was introduced. Rather than adding presidential leadership to the effort, however, the Clintons convened many stakeholders from the

insurance and business community to draft a proposal for the Clinton Health Plan, leaving it up to them to form a consensus. The resulting 1,342 page bill was filled with contradictions from stakeholders and could not even get out of committee in Congress [10]. The single payer bill (H. R. 1200), on the other hand, attracted the largest number of supporters in Congress, was the only competing bill to clear committee, but was soon marginalized by lobbyists and ridiculed by the major corporate media as too "extreme" or "utopian" [11].

2. Lessons We Can Learn from Past Failures of Health Care Reform

Although the details vary, there are common threads leading to defeats in each of those cases that are still with us. As we try to go forward with more effective reform today, we can learn from these patterns from the opposition [12].

1. *Turning to the stakeholders, who themselves created the system's problems, for recommended solutions, does not work.*

    The Clinton Health Plan in 1993-1994 is a classic example of this point. The Health Care Task Force convened by Hillary Clinton, representing mainly stakeholders in the insurance and business communities, worked behind closed doors while seeking little or no input from health policy and public health circles. In 2009, the Obama administration fell into the same trap by starting to negotiate deals with stakeholder industries, thereby reducing prospects for real reform.

2. *The more complex a bill becomes, in an effort to respond to conflicting political interests, the more its legislative and public support erodes.*

    Compromise begets more compromise, thereby adding to the cumulative complexity of any proposal and limiting the effectiveness of any reform bill if it ever does get passed. That occurred with the run-up to the Affordable Care Act during 2009-2010, ending with a final 2,000-plus page Senate bill. That stands in sharp contrast to the successful passage of the Canada Health Act of 1984, defined by five basic principles—public administration, comprehensiveness, universality, portability, and accessibility—in only several pages [13].

3. *Strong presidential leadership from the start and throughout the legislative process is critical to enactment of health care reform.*

   Social security could never have been enacted in 1935 had FDR not provided strong leadership all the way to its enactment. History would have been very different had President Bill Clinton given his support to the McDermott-Conyers-Wellstone single payer bill in 1993-1994 instead of his failed Clinton Health Plan [14].

4. *Corporate power in our enormous medical-industrial complex trumps the democratic process.*

   Corporate stakeholders and their well-funded lobbyists are expert at traveling the revolving door between industry, government and K Street in pursuit of their own self-interest. Because stake challengers are in such a comparatively weakened position, independent and non-partisan advocates of the public interest need to be actively involved throughout the political process for a reform proposal to be adopted.

5. *The "mainstream" media are not mainstream at all, and have conflicts of interest based on their close ties to corporate stakeholders in the status quo.*

   Because the major media conglomerates are businesses that rely on advertising revenue and the goodwill of the business community [15], there are many close and invisible ties between corporate health care interests and the media. For example, General Electric is heavily invested in medical and insurance industries. It also owns NBC, which has slammed universal health care [16]. During the 1993-1994 reform attempt, ABC's World News Tonight mentioned the single payer proposal just once, and some TV station managers admitted their reluctance to run ads favoring single payer in order to avoid antagonizing the insurance industry [17].

6. *We can count on opponents to use fear mongering to distort the health care debate.*

   This practice goes way back in time, even to 1912, when a proposal for NHI was cast by its opponents as "the nation's greatest international threat—that it was a plot by the German emperor to take over the United States" [18]. Fast forward to the 1990s, when the health insurance industry raised doubts about the Clinton Health Plan through Harry and Louise, the fictional couple who worried that the plan would hurt the middle class more than help them [18]. And then on to the debate during 2009-2010, when conservatives and their allies launched a well-funded and coordinated campaign against health care reform, with messages ranging from the government is the enemy to the superiority of free markets to fix problems. The health insurance industry created a group, Health Care America, in an effort to discredit Michael Moore's movie, Sicko, and denigrate successful health care systems, such as France and Canada, through disinformation [19].

Table 11.1 shows how distorted the vocabulary had become during those times [20], while Figure 11.1 captures these efforts as the Great Noise Machine of the right [21].

Table 11.1. The vocabulary of health care

WHAT IS SAID	WHAT IS HEARD
Universal health care	Socialized medicine
Health reform	Washington takeover
Individual mandate	Coerced health insurance
Shared responsibility	Higher taxes
Comparative effectiveness	Rationing of health care research
Public option	Predatory government, unfair competition
Advanced directives	Death panels
Health care exchange	Restricted choice
Medicare savings	Curtailed benefits, higher premiums
Rising numbers of uninsured	More "young invincibles"

Source: Wolf, S. (Ed.) Health debate or Health Charade? *Health Letter* 25(10)11, October, 2009.

7. *Centrist middle of the road reform proposals for health care are bound to fail.*

Such proposals tend to be watered down by responding to concerns from both the right and left to the point of being ineffective as reform proposals.

8. *Framing the basic issues in the health care reform debate has been inadequate; the alternatives have been controlled by the special interests resisting reform so they will win.*

   The major question in health care reform boils down to whether we should retain a for-profit inefficient, unaffordable, unreliable and wasteful multi-payer financing system or replace it with not-for-profit, public financing coupled with a private delivery system. Those stark contrasts cut to the core differences of the policy alternatives, and have yet to be presented that way in the health care debate.

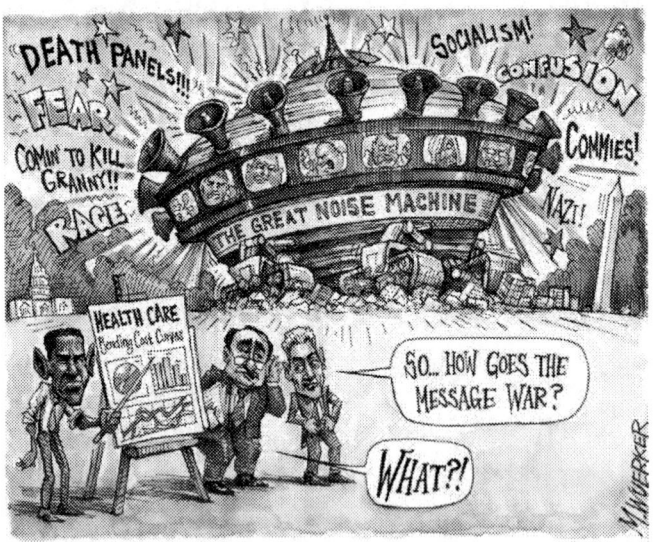

Matt Wuerker Editorial Cartoon used with permission of Matt Wuerker and the Cartoonist Group. All rights reserved.

Figure 11.1. The great noise machine.

9. *History repeats itself, and we don't learn from past mistakes.*

   As we look back upon failed efforts to reform health care over more than a century, it becomes obvious that the reasons for failure are repetitive, especially how corporate opponents of reform succeed in framing the debate to their self-interest and the corporate media are not held to account for their conflicts of interest. Winston Churchill has noted this chronic problem in these words:

Americans will always do the right thing—after they exhaust all the alternatives.

3. Obstacles Facing Reform Attempts Today

We will return to discuss in Chapter 13 the only reform alternative that can provide universal coverage to health care for all Americans — single payer NHI. We will need to learn the lessons described above if we are to see this increasingly urgent need met through a fair and responsible political process. As the economic stakes have become so high for the involved corporate stakeholders, however, we can expect an intense battle between them and the public interest once again.

While it is hard to predict the makeup of Congress after the 2022 and 2024 election cycles, we can anticipate that this kind of landscape will again be in play, by now an all too familiar battleground.

3.1. Activated Opposition from the Medical-Industrial Complex

Figure 11.2 illustrates the entangled complexity of the strangle-hold over reform proposals that would likely be brought to bear again this time in their corporate self-interest.

Corporate defenders already lie in wait for the next battle, as shown by these examples:

- Leading insurance, hospital and pharmaceutical lobbyists have formed the America's Health Care Future to defeat single payer Medicare for All through heavy lobbying and a targeted disinformation campaign [22].
- Figure 11.3 illustrates how many members of Congress can leave health reform behind by partaking of campaign contributions from a well-funded health insurance industry.
- Wendell Potter, former executive with Cigna and author of *Deadly Spin: An Insurance Company Insider Speaks Out on How Corporate PR is Killing Health Care and Deceiving Americans*, has analyzed the propaganda campaign by the private health insurance industry in

spreading Fear, Uncertainty and Doubt (FUD) about Medicare for All in these ways:

> "—FUD: We can't afford Medicare for All. TRUTH: We can't afford the status quo.
> —FUD: Medicare for all will be too disruptive. TRUTH: Insurers and employers have been disrupting Americans for years to protect profits.
> —FUD: Americans don't want 'one size fits all' health care. They want choice.
> TRUTH: It is not the choice of health insurance plans that Americans want, it is the choice of doctors and hospitals.
> —FUD: Americans who have employer-sponsored health insurance love it and don't want anything to replace it. TRUTH: The truth is that Americans are spending more and more every year for their employer-sponsored coverage and getting less and less value for the money they and their employers are spending on it" [23].

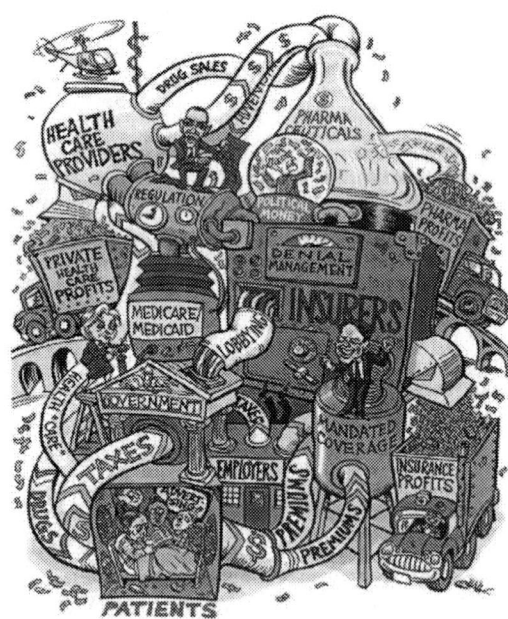

Source: Reprinted with permission of Tom Chalkley and *Tikkun Magazine*.

Figure 11.2. The octopus squeezing congressional debate and action.

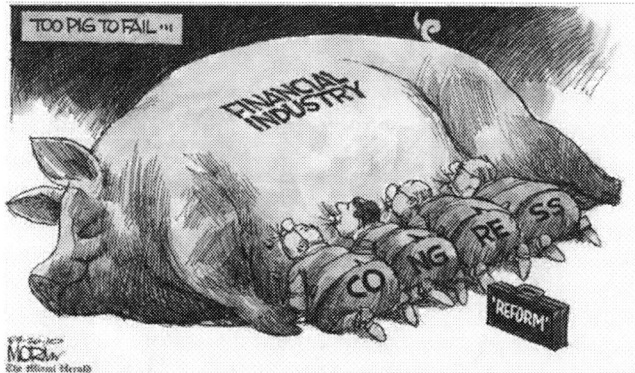

Source: Potter, W. I used to be a propagandist for insurance companies. Learn the four truths the insurance industry doesn't want Americans to see. *Tarbell,* April 30, 2019.

Figure 11.3. Too pig to fail.

- A GOP outside group aligned with then Senate Majority Leader Mitch McConnell (R- KY) launched a multi-million-dollar ad campaign against Medicare for All targeting legislators in both parties with campaign contributions as they spread doubts about Medicare for All, such as Rep. Cheri Bustos (D-IL), the chair of the Democratic Congressional Campaign Committee (DCCC), who thereafter said that the costs would be "scary" [24].
- More recently, in a unified display to protect the existing system from major reform, a coalition including hospitals (the American Hospital Association and the Federation of American Hospitals), insurers (America's Health Insurance Plans), and physicians (the American Medical Association) have joined together under a banner that "Americans deserve a stable health care market that provides access to high-quality care and affordable coverage for all," disingenuously without admitting that our existing system can never provide all of that [25].

3.2. A Swinging Revolving Door

The blatant conflicts of interest through the revolving door between industry, government and K Street influence resultant legislation, even to the point of control. That occurred with Elizabeth "Liz" Fowler's recurrent trip through the revolving door back in 2009-2010 with the ACA and now today with whatever legislation may come forward in the next session of Congress. As Chief Health Counsel to then Senate Finance Committee Chairman Max Baucus, she is credited with having crafted the ACA to the interests of the private insurance industry while that committee expelled and had arrested single payer advocates from the Senate's hearing room [26]. She had been vice president of public policy and external affairs at Wellpoint, which became Anthem of the Big 5 health insurers. Those close ties to industry did not receive much attention by the mainstream media [27].

After that tour in the public sector, she left Capitol Hill for a senior-level position dealing with "global health policy" at Johnson & Johnson's governmental affairs and policy group [28]. Now she is back, heading up the Center for Medicare and Medicaid Innovation (CMMI) within the Center for Medicare and Medicaid Services, where she keeps working to ward off not-for-profit NHI by continuing to explore ways in which private insurance can "save money" through already discredited "value-based payment" systems [29]. Her goal this time—to further expand Medicare Advantage, with all its methods of profiteering, including through DCE's (direct contract entities) [30]. Again, this conflict of interest was largely overlooked by the mainstream media. Figure 11.4 shows how the revolving door works back and forth from the public and private sectors [31].

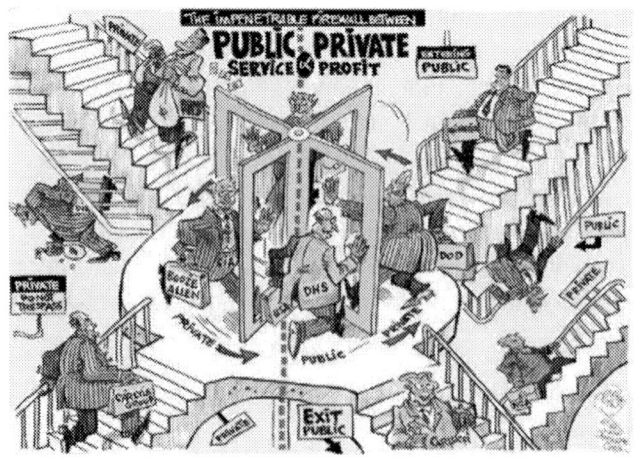

Source: Moyers, B, Winship, M. Washington's revolving door is hazardous to our health. *Common Dreams,* December 14.

Figure 11.4. The private-public revolving door as it perpetuates corporate interests.

3.3. Pressure Groups from Both Political Parties

Splits within both major political parties, together with each divided faction pressing its case in congressional debate, can readily block advancement of a bipartisan reform proposal. Moreover, the warring sides during that process are especially vulnerable to a quid pro quo from campaign contributions from industry. The words of William Greider, well known political journalist and author of the 1992 book, *Who Will Tell the People: The Betrayal of American Democracy,* apply today:

> *Government has been disabled or captured by the formidable powers of private enterprise and concentrated wealth. Self-governing rights that representative democracy conferred on citizens are now usurped by the overbearing demands of corporate and financial interests. Collectively, the corporate sector has its arms around both political parties, the financing of political careers, the production of policy agendas and propaganda of influential think tanks, and control of most major media* [32].

Ralph Nader adds this further perspective:

> *Corporate welfare is larger, more varied, and more automatic than ever. Subsidies, handouts, giveaways, and bailouts are now routinely enacted by little-challenged, government-guaranteed capitalism at the federal and state levels* [33].

Conclusion

Based on the foregoing, it's a wonder that any legislation gets enacted by Congress with anything close to its original intent. But as the stakes rise with an increasingly dysfunctional health care system, these obstacles must be recognized and dealt with in the public interest without being hidden in the underbrush. It is now time to move to the last three chapters, where we will describe the battle between "free market" proposals from the private sector vs. universal coverage through single payer Medicare for All.

References

[1] Giroux, HA. Surviving the second Gilded Age. *Truthout*, December 13, 2011.
[2] Burrow, JG. *AMA: Voice of American Medicine*. Baltimore. *Johns Hopkins Press*, 1963, 144.
[3] Compulsory health insurance. *JAMA* 74 (18): 1276, 1920.
[4] Somers, AR, Somers, HM. *Health and Health Care: Policies in Perspective*. Germantown, MD: *Aspen Systems Corp*, 1977.
[5] Rovner, J. In health care debate, fear trumps logic. *NPR,* August 28, 2009.
[6] Starr, P. *The Social Transformation of American Medicine*. New York. *Basic Books*, 1982.
[7] Ibid # 7.
[8] Schiltz, ME. *Public Attitudes Toward Social Security, 1935-1965*. Research report no. 33. Washington, D.C. Social Security Administration, Office of Research and Statistics, 1970: 136-139.
[9] Iglehart, JK. Compromise seems unlikely on three major insurance plans. *National Journal Reports*, May 11, 1974L 6L 700-707.
[10] Gordon, C. *The Clinton Health Care Plan: Dead on Arrival*. Westfield, NJ: *Open Magazine Pamphlet Series*, 1995.
[11] Brundin, J. How the U.S. press covers the Canadian health care system. *Intl J Health Services* 23 (2): 275-277, 1993.
[12] Geyman, JP. *America's Mighty Medical-Industrial Complex: Negative Impacts and Positive Solutions*. Friday Harbor, WA. *Copernicus Healthcare*, 2021, pp.218-219.
[13] Armstrong, P, Armstrong, H. *Universal Health Care: What the United States Can Learn from the Canadian Experience*. New York. *The New Press*, 1998: 6-32.
[14] Ibid # 8.
[15] Nader, R. *Crashing the Party: Taking on the Corporate Government in an Age of Surrender*. New York. *St. Martin's Griffin*, 2002.
[16] Hart, P, Naurecker, J. NBC slams universal health care. *EXTRA!*, December 2002, p. 4.
[17] Navarro, V. Why Congress did not enact health care reform. *J Health Polit Policy Law* 20: 196-199, 1995.
[18] Ibid # 5.
[19] Potter, W. Rally against Wall Street's health care takeover. *Truthout*, September 1, 2009.
[20] Wolf, S (Ed.). Health debate or health charade? *Health Letter* 25 (10): 11, October, 2009.
[21] Baker, D. The public plan option and the big government conservatives. *The Progressive Populist* 15: 18, October 15, 2009, p. 12.
[22] Fang, L, Surgey, N. Lobbyist documents reveal health care industry battle plan against Medicare for All. *The Intercept*, November 20, 2018.
[23] Potter, W. I used to be a propagandist for insurance companies. Learn the four truths the insurance industry doesn't want Americans to see. *Tarbell*, April 30, 2019.
[24] Potter, W. Democrats on the take: New DCCC chair is a best friend of health insurers. *Tarbell*, March 15, 2019.

[25] Abelson, R. Broad coalition of health industry groups calls for Obamacare expansion. *New York Times*, February 10, 2021.
[26] Editorial. Puppets in Congress. *New York Times*, November 17, 2009: A 1.
[27] Connor, K. Chief health aide to Baucus is former WellPoint executive. *Eyes on the Ties Blog,* September 1, 2009.
[28] Light, J. Stories from Washington's revolving door. *Moyers & Company*, December 14, 2012.
[29] Tillow, K. Liz Fowler is back! And she's writing U.S. health policy again. *CounterPunch*, June 7, 2021.
[30] Gilfillan, R, Berwick, DM. Medicare Advantage & DCEs: How corporate investors deplete Medicare. *Health Affairs Blog*, September 27 & 28, 2021.
[31] Moyers, B, Winship, M. Washington's revolving door is hazardous to our health. *Common Dreams*, December 14, 2012.
[32] Greider, W. The end of New Deal liberalism. *The Nation*, January 5, 2011.
[33] Nader, R. In the Public Interest: Think big to overcome losing big to corporatism. *The Progressive Populist*, February 15, 2022.

Part 3: Major Opposing Future Scenarios for Reform of Health Care

> *To choose a more egalitarian society requires a robust democratic politics. When democratic counterweights are weak, the power of money prevails... Leave health care to the market, and some people will die on the street for want of medical attention, the sick will be ejected from health plans, doctors will be turned against patients, and insurance companies and magnates will grow very rich*[1].

—Robert Kuttner, Co-founder of *The American Prospect* and author of the important 1999 book, *Everything for Sale: The Virtues and Limits of Markets*

> *The hard fact is that the way to health-care reform in the USA requires political activism of the most basic kind, something that is far beyond the comfort zone of many health professionals*[2].

—Dr. David Blumenthal, President of The Commonwealth Fund, and Dr. Margaret Hamburg, President of the American Association for the Advancement of Science

---

[1] Kuttner, R. *The Squandering of America: How the Failure of Our Politics Undermines Our Prosperity.* New York. *Alfred A Knopf,* 2007, p.10.

[2] Blumenthal, D, Hamburg, M. U.S. health and health care are a mess: Now what? *The Lancet,* February 11, 2021.

Chapter 12

"Free Market" Alternatives without Fundamental Reform

> *I find little evidence anywhere that market forces, bluntly used, that is, consumer choice among an array of products with competitors fighting it out, leads to a health care system you want and need. In the U.S. competition has become toxic: it is a major reason for our duplicative, supply-driven, fragmented health care system* [1].

—Don Berwick, M.D., former administrator of the Centers for Medicare and Medicaid Services and founder of the Institute for Healthcare Improvement.

The above statement 14 years ago by a health policy expert with long experience in administration, stands today as a cutting-edge truth that continues to undermine U.S. health care. The goals of this chapter are: (1) to summarize the extent of how broken the U.S. health care system has become; (2) to briefly consider how "free market" reform theories of health care and insurance continue to undermine system reform; and (3) to consider three "free market" reform proposals.

1. The Broken Health Care System in the U.S.

Table 12.1 gives us a quick overview of system problems today in the U.S. This list is virtually the same as 20 years ago, completely resistant to any reform efforts, such as the Affordable Care Act of 2010. With that broad overview, let's focus on one individual with a common serious chronic disease to see how affordable the ACA has made health care.

> *Alec R. Smith, 26, aged off from his mother's health insurance plan on his birthday. He had been on insulin for years for Type I diabetes. He and his mother explored options over the three months before his birthday. His annual income as a restaurant manager was about $35,000, too high to qualify for Medicaid and also too high to be eligible*

for subsidies under Minnesota's ACA insurance marketplace. The plan they found [was unaffordable with] a monthly premium of $450 and an annual deductible of $7,600. He hoped to afford his $1,300 monthly bill for diabetes supplies (mostly for insulin) by getting a part-time job. But he died of diabetic ketoacidosis a month later [in 2018], just three days before payday, having apparently rationed his insulin, with an empty insulin syringe at his side [2].

Table 12.1. Major problems of U.S. health care

1. Uncontrolled inflation of health care costs and prices.
2. Growing crisis in unaffordability of health care now extending to middle class.
3. Decreasing access to care.
4. Increasing health disparities.
5. Rising rates of uninsured and underinsured.
6. Discontinuity and turnover of insurance coverage.
7. Variable, often poor quality of care.
8. High rates of inappropriate and unnecessary care with physician induced demand.
9. Administrative complexity, profiteering and waste of private health insurers.
10. Decreased choice of hospital and physician in managed care programs.
11. Erosion of safety net programs.
12. Declining primary care base.
13. Inadequate national system for assessment of new medical technologies, insufficient use of cost-effectiveness analysis.
14. Lax federal regulation of drug, medical device, and dietary supplement industries.
15. Market-based system more accountable to corporate stakeholders and investors than to patients.

That single vignette exposes the complexity and irrationality of our public-private multi-payer insurance "system," together with the total failure of the ACA to contain prices for an old and common medication. The cost of a single vial of insulin in 2018 was more than $250, and most patients use two to four vials each month [3]. Boston-based Sanofi, a major pharmaceutical company producing insulin, has marked up prices for its insulin products by as much as 4,500 percent over the estimated cost of producing a single vial of insulin. With insulin no longer affordable for many patients with Type I diabetes, many others are dying after trying to ration their insulin. Grieving mothers led a march against Sanofi in 2019, carrying the ashes of their dead children and demanding that the company cut its prices [4].

Bringing those prices up to date in 2022, the cost of insulin has tripled in the U.S. over the last 10 years, with the price for a single vial still ranging up to $1,000. Three drug makers control almost 100% of the U.S. market, of life-saving importance to the 7 million Americans requiring its use. One in four of those 7 million ration insulin because of its high costs. The Inflation Reduction Act, passed in 2022, will help to make insulin more affordable by capping its monthly cost at $35 starting in 2023. [5].

Although unaffordability of health care is just one of the 15 major system problems shown in Table 12.1, it impacts a larger spectrum of care, including decreased access and worse outcomes of care. Gallup polling in December 2021 found that almost one-third of Americans said that they had skipped medical care in the previous three months due to cost; even 1 in 5 households earning more than $120,000 a year said the same thing [6].

1.1. "Free Market" Reform Proposals

We continue to have wrongheaded theories of how market-based health care would save money for all concerned if we would just let the markets work their magic through supposed competition. That claim, of course, has long since been proven specious as inflation of health care prices and costs continue unchecked and as corporate profiteering continues on the backs of patients, their families, and taxpayers.

These are some of the main disproven theories that cry out for fundamental reform:

1. "The private sector is more efficient than the public sector."
2. "Based on moral hazard, patients will abuse the system and overuse health care unless restraints are put in their way—such as high deductibles and other forms of cost sharing."
3. "Unless restraints are placed on physicians, they will be irresponsible in ordering too many tests and treatments."
4. "Managed competition" will contain costs and ensure quality of care."
5. "Value-based payment systems will save money and improve quality of care for Medicare patients."

Experience and evidence over many years contradicts all of these assertions, as these points indicate:

1. The private sector is far less efficient than the public sector, as evidenced by private insurers' administrative overhead five to six times higher than that of traditional public Medicare and Medicaid [7, 8].
2. Instead of over-utilization of health care, we have under-utilization on the part of patients, but over-utilization by corporate interests. Ironically and never admitted by private insurers and their corporate allies, we have *over*-utilization through unnecessary tests and procedures through such means as up-coding scams and manipulation of the electronic health record. Up to one-third too much care is being delivered, much unnecessary and some even harmful [9], but moral hazard is not the cause of health care inflation.
3. Most physicians are responsible to their patients' needs, including being sensitive to their wallets, but corporate interests keep driving for higher profits. The increased bureaucracy separating physicians from their patients, requiring them to spend much of their practice time on dealing with insurers, is leading increasing numbers of physicians to burn out and retire early [10]. Profiteering by insurers, pharmacy benefit managers, and other corporate stakeholders are the main culprits for unaffordable health care costs, including setting prices, not physicians or patients.
4. Managed care programs run by large corporate managers for both privatized Medicare and Medicaid, far from saving money, generate high returns for CEOs and investors while often associated with under-treatment of patients and poor quality of care [11, 12].
5. "Value-based" payment systems conducted in recent years by the Centers for Medicare and Medicaid, have all failed to improve quality of care [13].

This observation back in 1984 by Lester Thurow, Ph.D., economist and former Dean of the MIT Sloan School of Management, has been proven by time and experience to be correct:

> *We are not real believers in the free-market mechanism unless we can honestly say that we would be willing to see some patients suffer the consequences if they could not afford an available treatment being provided to wealthier patients. If we cannot really accept that, then we simply will not let the market work when push comes to shove.*

Proponents of the market approach also forget that an egalitarian distribution of health care is one of the factors that creates social solidarity, a feeling of community and the non-monetary attachments that bind a society together. If health care is not part of the social glue that holds us together, what is?

Health care costs are being treated as if they were largely an economic problem, but they are not. To be solved, they will have to be treated as an ethical problem [14].

2. Three Major GOP Reform Proposals

2.1. Build on the Affordable Care Act (ACA)

While the ACA was a helpful incremental step in 2010 by bringing health insurance to 20 million more Americans and bringing back coverage for about 8 million people who had lost coverage during the pandemic, the case against building on it is compelling for these reasons:

- "It would still be just another Band-Aid on a broken system far short of universal coverage.
- It has failed to contain costs, and will continue to do so since a profiteering, inefficient private insurance industry is left in place.
- Insurance and health care will remain unaffordable and inaccessible for a large part of our population.
- COVID-19 care will not be fully covered.
- Continued inequities, with many Americans still delaying or foregoing essential care.
- Health insurance still pricey and volatile as employer-based coverage is further stressed.
- Regulation of network size has been inadequate, while insurers continue to game the system for profits.
- Many insurers abandon markets that are not sufficiently profitable, often with little advance notice.
- A continued Medicaid coverage gap exists in the 12 states that refused to expand Medicaid" [15].

Although almost 14 million more people have signed up for ACA coverage under the recently completed open-enrollment period [16], all of the above limits still apply to the lack of fundamental system reform 12 years after its passage.

2.2. Medicare for Some

These are incremental approaches, including lowering the age of Medicare eligibility to age 60, as advanced by the Biden administration, and a public option for sale alongside private plans on the ACA's exchanges as not-for-profit CO-OPs (Consumer Oriented and Operated Plans). It was hoped that the CO-OPs could compete with their for-profit counterparts, and lower their costs, but they were a dismal failure. Just 4 of the 23 CO-OPs established under the ACA survive today, down from a peak of 1 million enrollees in 2015 to just 150,000, and hardly meeting its goal to lower prices. These proposals again would be just more incremental Band-Aids on our sick system that would fail for these reasons:

- Increased administrative complexity, costs, bureaucracy and waste.
- Non-comprehensive benefits.
- Restricted access to care through private insurers' networks.
- Continued high deductibles and other forms of cost sharing.
- Would leave at least 15 to 20 million people still uninsured [17].

2.3. Privatized Medicare Advantage for All

As we have seen in earlier chapters, the increasing rolls of Medicare Advantage have been fueled by ongoing efforts by conservatives to further privatize Medicare. That pressure has even been continued by the Centers for Medicare and Medicaid Services under the Biden administration, as a left-over idea from the Trump administration.

The track record of Medicare Advantage, however, at once refutes the idea that it could reform our system to the advantage of all Americans. It has already failed to meet the needs of its enrollees for these kinds of reasons:

"Free Market" Alternatives without Fundamental Reform

- Lack of cost containment
- Large overpayments and federal tax subsidies.
- Profiteering on the backs of patients and tax payers.
- Administrative overhead five to six times higher than that of traditional Medicare.
- Restrictions of access, continuity and quality of enrollees' care.
- Continued lack of universal coverage [18].

Collectively, these so-called reform proposals, based on discredited theories by conservatives, are just incremental steps that would fall far short of what's needed to reform U.S. health care. Each would just add more patches that won't work any better than those shown in Figure 12.1 [19]. But they will receive strong support from many of today's corporate stakeholders profiteering from the "free market" status quo. As just one example, the American Hospital Association (AHA) has already been in bed with venture capital as a source of support, as are many of its member hospitals [20].

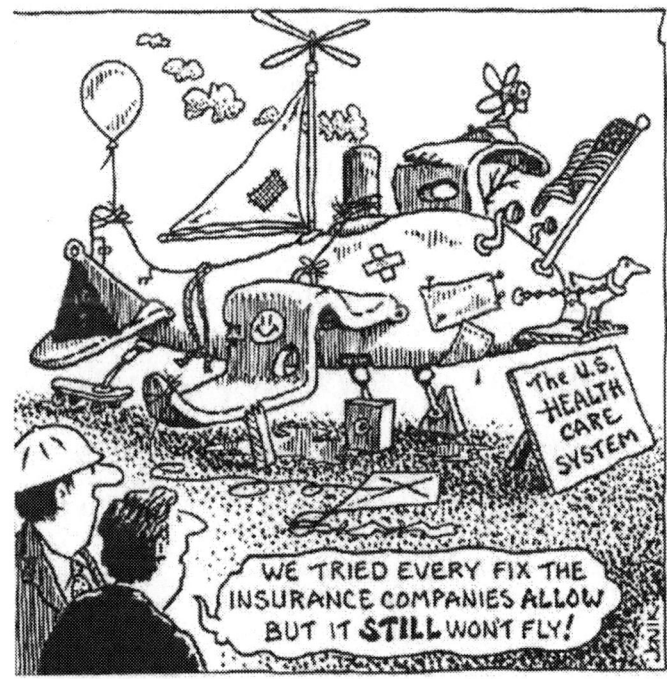

Source: Reprinted with permission of John Janik.

Figure 12.1. Incremental reform doesn't fix U.S. health care.

Conclusion

A fourth reform proposal—single payer Medicare for All—will be discussed in the next chapter, including its overwhelming advantages over any of the free market plans advanced by conservatives with their long track record of failure.

References

[1] Berwick, D. A transatlantic review of the NHS at 60. *British Medical Journal* 337 (7663): 212-214, 2008.
[2] Sable-Smith, B. Insulin's high cost leads to lethal rationing. *NPR*, September 1, 2018.
[3] Altman, D. It's not just the uninsured—it's also the cost of health care. *Axios*, August 20, 2018.
[4] Saini, V. As drug prices rise, is Boston's prosperity bases on a moral crime? *WBUR*, January 31, 2019.
[5] The Inflation Reduction Act lowers health care costs for millions of Americans. *Centers of Medicare and Medicaid Services*, October 5, 2022.
[6] Picchi, A. Surge in Americans skipping medical care due to cost, Gallup says. *CBS News*, December 14, 2021.
[7] Tillow, K. Beyond the Medicare Advantage scam. All Unions Committee for Single Payer Health Care. http://unionsforsinglepayer.org, September 14, 2020.
[8] Geruso, M, Layton, TL, Wallace, J. Are all managed care plans created equal? Evidence from random plan assignment in Medicaid, NBER Working Paper No. 27762, National Bureau of Economic Research, August 2020.
[9] Wenner, JB, Fisher, ES, Skinner, JS. Geography and the debate over Medicare reform. *Health Affairs Web Exclusive* W-103, February 13, 2002.
[10] Himmelstein, DU, Woolhandler, S. Comment on— Driving Physician Burnout: Corporate Takeover & Value-Based Care. *Health Justice Monitor*, September 7, 2021.
[11] Geyman, JP. *Shredding the Social Contract: The Privatization of Medicare.* Monroe, ME. *Common Courage Press*, 2006, p. 206.
[12] McCue, MJ, Bailit, MJ. Assessing the financial health of Medicaid managed care plans and the quality of care they provide. *The Commonwealth Fund*, June 15, 2011.
[13] Khullar, Dhruv, William L Schpero, Amelia M Bond, Yuting Qian, Lawrence P Casalino. Association between patient social risk and physician performance scores in the first year of the Merit-based Incentive Payment System. *JAMA*, September 8, 2020.
[14] Thurow, L. Sounding Board: Learning to say "No." *N Engl J Med* 311 (24): 1571, 1984.

[15] Geyman, JP. *America's Mighty Medical-Industrial Complex: Negative Impacts and Positive Solutions*. Friday Harbor, WA. *Copernicus Healthcare*, 2021, p. 264.
[16] Armour, S. Nearly 14 million enroll under ACA. *Wall Street Journal*, January 11, 2022: A 7.
[17] Himmelstein, DU, Woolhandler, S. The 'public option' on health care is a poison pill. *The Nation*, October 21, 2019.
[18] Geyman, JP. Privatized Medicare Advantage for All: The latest assault on U.S. health care. *Intl J Health Services*, October 27, 2021.
[19] Geyman, JP. *Do Not Resuscitate: Why the Health Insurance Industry Is Dying, and How We Must Replace It*. Monroe, ME. *Common Courage Press*, 2008, p. 137.
[20] Bannow, T. A hospital lobbying juggernaut makes an unlikely pivot into venture capital. *STAT +*, March 24, 2022.

Chapter 13

Universal Coverage through National Health Insurance

> *The wreckage of the New Deal regulatory model has allowed the hyper concentration of finance, with proliferation of business modes such as hedge funds and private equity that do little to help the real economy but allow astronomical incomes at the top as well as intensified turbulence of ordinary companies and workers. The financial collapse provided both a reason and an occasion for the Obama administration to perform Roosevelt-style surgery on Wall Street. But Obama's team settled for tinkering around the edges. High incomes are more highly concentrated than ever* [1].
>
> —Robert Kuttner, founder and coeditor of The American Prospect and author of the 2007 book, *Everything for Sale* and *the End of Laissez-Faire*

The foregoing chapters have shown that corporate stakeholders in our massive medical-industrial complex have created a dysfunctional health care non-system that meets their needs for large profits at the expense of patients, families, health professionals and taxpayers. Recurrent reform efforts over recent decades have failed to rein in private profiteering of what is now one-sixth of the nation's GDP. The goals of this chapter are (1) to lay out values for successful reform as have been demonstrated by the experience of other advanced nations over many years; (2) to summarize why the profiteering, private health insurance industry no longer meets the needs of the American people; (3) why it should be replaced by a single payer, not-for-profit system of national health insurance (NHI); and (4) to compare NHI with the three 'free market' proposals described in the last chapter, and briefly consider how it can be achieved through transition away from today's corporate control of health care.

1. Reform Based on Equity and a Service Ethic

Based on the experience of other advanced countries around the world over many years, these ten values can effectively serve as the basis for health care reform in the U.S.:

1. "Health care is a human right, as supported by moral, medical, economic, social and public health considerations.
2. Health care is an essential person-based and population-based service, not a commodity for sale to the highest bidder.
3. The prevailing ethic in health care should shift from a for-profit business "ethic" to an ethic of service.
4. Health care should be available to all based on medical need, not ability to pay.
5. Patients and families should have full choice of physician and hospital everywhere in the country.
6. Our delivery system should be readily accessible, reliable, and efficient.
7. Health insurance should be not-for-profit, with minimal administrative bureaucracy and waste.
8. Our financing system should share risk across the entire population in order to achieve the most affordable coverage.
9. Coverage decisions should be based on science, with the goal of efficacy, cost-effectiveness, and safety of treatments.
10. A reformed health care system should be based on the public interest, not the profit motives of today's medical-industrial complex" [2].

Howard Bauchner, M.D., editor of the *Journal of the American Medical Association* (*JAMA*) has thrown his full support to the importance of health care as a human right:

All physicians, including those who are members of Congress, other health care professionals, and professional societies (should) speak with a single voice and say that health care is a basic right for every person, and not a privilege to be available and affordable only for a majority [3].

2. Why the Failed Private Health Insurance Industry Should Be Replaced

The private health insurance industry has had a long run since its debut, as a not-for-profit Blue Cross plan in Texas in the 1930s, during the depths of the Great Depression. As described in Chapters 2 and 9, it served the public interest for many years after that. Beyond the 1960s, however, it became increasingly dominated by the primary goal to make money for corporations and their shareholders. Here are compelling reasons to replace it with a not-for-profit single payer system of national health insurance under Medicare for All [4]:

- Employer-sponsored insurance (ESI), its largest component from the beginning, is now too unreliable and volatile; in 2018, for example, 66 million Americans left or lost their jobs, with many not regaining insurance *if* they became re-employed [5].
- ESI restricts choice in many ways, including narrowing and ever-changing networks of physicians and hospitals.
- The average denial rate for in-network claims across the industry is 18 percent [6].
- Our current largely for-profit multi-payer financing system leaves about 28 million people uninsured and 87 million underinsured.
- A recent Public Citizen report found that the uninsured accounted for 40 percent of U.S. COVID-19 cases and one-third of its deaths, many of which could have been prevented by having insurance [7].
- ESI has become unaffordable for both workers and employers, especially small business that represents most businesses on Main Street; premiums and deductibles have soared far above workers' wages (Figure 9.1).
- Private health insurers game the system at enrollees' expense through deceptive marketing, cost sharing with ever rising deductibles and co-pays, and limited drug formularies.
- Cost sharing at the point of care leads to many patients delaying or foregoing essential care. (Figure 2.3).
- Privatized Medicare Advantage has bloated administrative costs 5 to 6 times higher than that of traditional public Medicare.
- Private insurers often exit unprofitable markets with little advance notice, leaving enrollees in the lurch.

- Profiteering, even during the COVID pandemic, racking up high revenue while tens of millions of Americans were losing their jobs and ESI [8].
- Profiteering on privatized public programs—Medicare and Medicaid—through overpayments (Figure 2.1), even while receiving federal subsidies averaging $685 billion a year [9].

Table 9.2 summarizes the main reasons that call for retiring a failing private health insurance industry with its multi-payer financing system [10]. Table 13.1 shows how traditional American values are consistent with and supportive of getting rid of multi-payer financing of U.S. health care.

Table 13.1. Alternative financing systems and American values

TRADITIONAL VALUE	Single-Payer	Multi-Payer
Efficiency	↑	↓
Choice	↑	↓
Affordability	↑	↓
Actuarial value	↑	↓
Fiscal responsibility	↑	↓
Equitable	↑	↓
Accountable	↑	↓
Integrity	↑	↓
Sustainable	↑	↓

3. National Health Insurance with Single-Payer Public Financing

Single-payer, not-for-profit Medicare for All is the only effective way to reform our dysfunctional system by addressing its inadequate access, unaffordable prices and costs, unacceptable quality, and widespread disparities and inequities. There is already a bill in the House of Representatives— H. R. 1976— which, if and when enacted would bring:

Universal Coverage through National Health Insurance 139

- Universal coverage for comprehensive benefits through a new system of national health insurance for all U.S. residents, based on medical need, not ability to pay.
- Full choice of hospitals, physicians, and other health professionals anywhere in the country.
- Elimination of cost-sharing at the point of care, such as deductibles, co-pays and pre-authorization of services.
- Administrative simplification with efficiencies and cost containment through large-scale cost controls, including (a) negotiated fee schedules for physicians and other health professionals, who will remain in private practice; (b) global annual budgeting of hospitals and other facilities; and (c) bulk purchasing of drugs and medical devices.
- Sharing of risk for the costs of illness and accidents across our entire population of 330 million Americans.
- Cost savings that enable universal coverage through a not-for-profit single-payer financing system.

Gerald Friedman, Ph.D., Professor of Economics at the University of Massachusetts Amherst and author of the book, *The Case for Medicare for All*, estimates that more than $1 trillion would have been saved had it been in place in 2019 (Figure 13.1) [11].

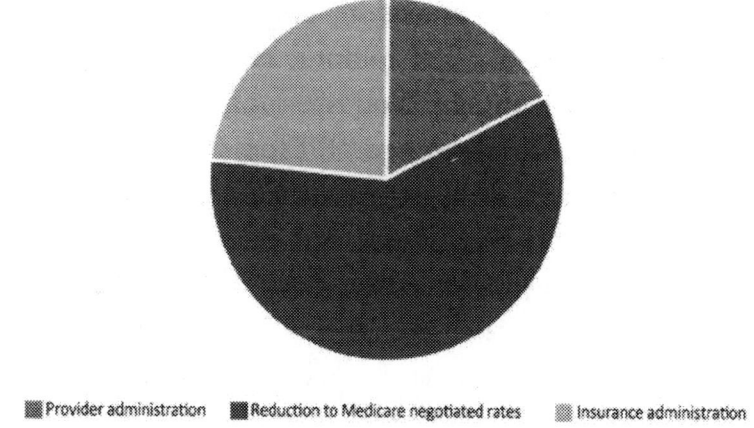

Provider administration ■ Reduction to Medicare negotiated rates ■ Insurance administration

Source: Friedman, G. "The Case for Medicare for All." Medford, MA, *Polity Press*, 2020, p. 62.

Figure 13.1. Medicare for all savings compared to current system, 2019.

4. Comparision of Four Reform Alternatives

Tables 13.2 and 13.3 compare the three for-profit private "free market" reform alternatives with single-payer not-for-profit Medicare for All in terms of values and evidence, respectively [12].

Table 13.2. Value-based comparison of four reform alternatives

	ACA	PUBLIC OPTION	MEDICARE ADVANTAGE FOR ALL	MEDICARE FOR ALL
Health care a human right	No	No	No	Yes
Commodity for sale?	Yes	Yes	Yes	No
Profit vs. service ethic	Profit	Profit	Profit	Service
Full choice of physician & hospital	No	No	No	Yes
Accessable, reliable, efficient?	No	No	No	Yes
Not for profit, reduced waste?	No	No	No	Yes
Population-based, shared risk?	No	No	No	Yes
Science-based?	No	No	No	Yes
Common good, public interest?	No	No	No	Yes

Table 13.3. Evidence-based comparison of four reform alternatives

	ACA	PUBLIC OPTION	MEDICARE ADVANTAGE FOR ALL	MEDICARE FOR ALL
Access	Restricted	Restricted	Restricted	Unrestricted
Choice	Restricted	Restricted	Restricted	Unrestricted
Cost containment	Never	Never	Never	Yes
Quality of care	Unacceptable	Unacceptable	Unacceptable	Improved
Bureaucracy	Large, wasteful	Large, wasteful	Large, wasteful	Much reduced
Universal coverage	Never	Never	Never	Yes
Accountability	No	No	No	Yes
Sustainability	No	No	No	Yes

Adam Gaffney, past president of Physicians for a National Health Program and author of *To Heal Humankind: The Right to Health in History*, brings this important perspective to the urgent need to rebuild our health care system for best access and quality of patient care for all Americans, not corporate and Wall Street profits:

> *We need to envision a health system where the distribution of infrastructure and resources is not left to the dictates of the market, but rationally planned according to the needs of communities—and the certainty of future disasters. It requires discarding the false promise of anarchical medical competition as the salve of our healthcare cost crisis* [13].

Drs. Himmelstein and Woolhandler, co-founders of Physicians for a National Health Program (PNHP) in the late 1980s and steadfast leaders of the health reform movement since then, have recently pointed out in a landmark article this glaring obstacle today—how can you implement NHI when most of the health care system is already owned and operated by a mega-merged, Wall Street backed profiteering corporatized industry? They recommend this excellent strategy to make a transition over to NHI:

> *A transition to public, community-based ownership—a reform model generally labeled National Health Service (NHS), in contrast to NHI—seems the most appropriate solution, especially since taxpayers have directly or indirectly bankrolled the construction of most hospitals and other facilities. Such an NHS should have federal funding and oversight, similar to the Veterans Health Administration—a publicly owned and operated health system that delivers high quality of care at lower cost than the private sector* [14].

They have also added this further important insight:

> *There is absolutely no question that we have an expensive but highly flawed, fragmented health care financing system that is not delivering value, especially considering the numbers that are uninsured and underinsured. We now have extensive data demonstrating that we can correct this by simply enacting a single payer system, an improved Medicare for All.*
>
> *What we have failed to address is the adverse financial consequences of corporate dominance and private equity takeovers of our health care delivery system. In supporting a public health care financing system to serve us all, shouldn't we also be supporting a delivery system dedicated to the public? How better could we do this than by establishing community ownership? It would be nice to have our owners—ourselves—primarily interested in our health care, rather than be primarily interested in acquiring our money.*

> *Health care reform must address who owns health care, not only who pays the bill. Taxpayers' and patients' dollars have paid to build the U.S. health care system: the public must reclaim ownership of it. Following Scotland's National Health Service, we should recast patients (in partnership with health care personnel) as owners of the health care system, not its customers* [15].

Conclusion

The above concept shines a new bright light on the daunting challenge to change ownership of our corporatized health care system to communities and patients. How to get there from here becomes the big question, which requires us to consider the forces for and against this kind of fundamental reform, as we will in the next and last chapter.

References

[1] Kuttner, R. Will Biden be radical enough? *The American Prospect*, March/April 2021, 5.

[2] Geyman, JP. *America's Mighty Medical-Industrial Complex: Negative Impacts and Positive Solutions*. Friday Harbor, WA. *Copernicus Healthcare*, 2021, pp 235-239.

[3] Bauchner, H. Health care in the United States: A right or a privilege. *JAMA* 317 (1): 323, January 3, 2017.

[4] Geyman, JP. The private health insurance industry: Should it be eliminated? *CounterPunch*, March 5, 2021.

[5] Bruenig, M. People lose their employer-sponsored insurance constantly. *People's Advocacy Project*, April 4, 2019.

[6] Silvers, JB. This is the most realistic path to Medicare for All. *New York Times*, October 16, 2019.

[7] Kemp, E. *Unprepared for COVID-19: How the Pandemic Makes the Case for Medicare for All*. Washington, D.C. *Public Citizen*, March 16, 2021.

[8] Appleby, J, Findley, S. Health insurers prosper as COVID-19 deflates demand for elective treatments. *Kaiser Health News*, April 28, 2020.

[9] Ockerman, E. It costs $685 billion a year to subsidize U.S. health insurance. *Bloomberg News*, May 23, 2018.

[10] Geyman, JP. *Do Not Resuscitate: Why the Health Insurance Industry Is Dying, and How We Must Replace It*. Monroe, ME. *Common Courage Press*, 2008, p. 112.

[11] Friedman, G. *The Case for Medicare for All*. Medford, MA. *Polity Press*, 2020, p. 62.

[12] Geyman, JP. *Transformation of U.S. Health Care: 1960-2020: One Family Physician's Journey*. Friday Harbor, WA. *Copernicus Healthcare*, 2022, p. 160.
[13] Gaffney, A. Bring back health planning. *Dissent Magazine*, Summer 2020.
[14] Himmelstein, David U, Steffie Woolhandler, Adam Gaffney, Don McCanne and John Geyman. Medicare is not enough: Communities, not corporations, should own our most vital health care assets. *The Nation*, March 31, 2022.
[15] Himmelstein, DU, Woolhandler, S. *Health Justice Monitor*, March 31, 2022.

Chapter 14

"Free Market" Profiteering vs. Not-for-Profit Patient Care: Which Will Prevail in 2040?

> *Economic elites and organized groups representing business interests not only exert substantial impact, but their policy positions tend to be exactly the opposite of those of non-influential ordinary citizens* [1].
>
> —Martin Gilens, Ph.D. and Benjamin Page, Ph.D., Professors of Political Science at Princeton University and Northwestern University, respectively

The above quote is the conclusion drawn by two professors after analyzing a massive data set concerning the impacts of different groups on government policy in the U.S. They found broad bipartisan support for health care reform that was then cancelled out during the political process when large amounts of corporate money and lobbyists descended on Congress. All this is recounted by Dr. John Abramson in his 2022 book, *Sickening: How Big PhRMA Broke American Health Care and How We Can Repair It.*

That brings to light a key factor relating to whether and how we can reform our health care system given the political forces fighting for the status quo. This chapter has four goals: (1) to ask whether it is possible or already too late to get U.S. health care out from under its corporate umbrella of profiteering rather than service; (2) to consider reasons to be pessimistic about reform; (3) to consider reasons to be optimistic about reform; and (4) to discuss what the likely outcome will be by 2040 after the political battle over U.S. health care has evolved.

1. Is It Already too Late to Right the Health Care Ship?

One could come to that conclusion since the corporate structure in health care has become so well established and successful from a revenue building standpoint to become one-sixth of the nation's GDP. Further, we have to admit that medical organizations have been, with some exceptions, missing in action as corporate money has taken over their profession.

Peter Swenson, Ph.D., Professor of Political Science at Yale University and author of the 2021 book, *Disorder: A History of Reform, Reaction, and Money in American Medicine,* has brought us a disappointing story of how the medical profession has failed to confront its loss of professionalism while being bought off by corporate and Wall Street money. In the early years since its founding in 1847, the American Medical Association (AMA) took the high ground concerning conflicts of interest. It then held that "holding a patent for any drug or surgical advice was "derogatory to professional character" for doctors; accepting money to shill for industrial patent holders was a breach of ethics" [2].

Here are some of the lowlights as traced by Dr. Swenson of the AMA's deviation since then from its earlier ethical standards:

- Starting in the 1920s, organized medicine, including hundreds of specialty societies, discarded this staunch defiance of commercialism for wary collaboration and ultimately a full embrace of support from the pharmaceutical and medical device industries.
- In the 1950s, the AMA and the drug industry became fully enmeshed. JAMA relaxed its control on advertising to increase its revenue.
- In the early 1960s, 17 of the largest drug firms gave nearly $1 million to the AMA's lobbying firm to help it fight Medicare, in part out of fear of federal controls on drug pricing.
- In 1971, the AMA dropped from its ethical code its historic disapproval of medicine patents held by physicians. The next year, it shut down its semi-independent Council on Drugs that had issued advice on hundreds of products on the market to help clinicians separate good from useless—or worse—medications.
- In 1973, John Adriani, the chair of the now-disbanded council, indignantly explained to Congress that the AMA was "captive of, and beholden to, the pharmaceutical industry."
- In the last 40 years, specialty societies have eclipsed the AMA in overall importance and political muscle; they keep secret their sources of funding, but it is estimated that they receive almost 80 percent of their revenue from industry [3].

Dr. George Lundberg, Editor of the *Journal of the American Medical Association* for 17 years from 1982 to 1999, was a critic of the corporatization of medicine. He fought against the lack of equity in access to health care and the growing power of the private health insurance industry. He had this to say about reform and the future of health insurance in his 2000 book *Severed Trust: Why American Medicine Hasn't Yet Been Fixed:*

> *The probable scenario is that a government program, similar to Medicare, will be established for all U.S. residents within a decade or two. The push will come not from liberal legislators but rather from the flame-out of insurance companies or from employer support for a national system. Unless insurance companies miraculously exercise self-discipline, they will cherry-pick themselves out of business ... No country has achieved universal health insurance voluntarily. It must be mandatory* [4].

Here are several negative descriptions of changes in the health care landscape over the last 40 years as sent to me in response to my recent article in *Pharos*, "The business 'ethic' vs. service ethic in U.S. health care: Which will prevail"? [5]

- Family medicine residency graduate in 1970 who was a rural family physician for 27 years in eastern Oregon, followed by administration with insurance contractors:

> *I watched this start happening decades ago and each year it gets worse. This is very sad for U.S. patients and for U.S. docs as well. The profession has sold its soul to the devil for ever increasing income which does not buy happiness. Witness so many docs planning on retiring in the next couple of years.*

- Retired nephrologist after 50 years of practice in an academic hospital in Pennsylvania:

> *I experienced much of what you discussed [in the Pharos article]. Now my hospital is all for the dollars and has been refigured so it refused to take on an academic nephrologist and her fellows. Our group would publish and present work on CAPD as well as papers on other research topics. No more. Thanks for your insights and truth telling.*

- Academic family physician and ethicist in medical schools in Michigan and later Texas:

> *One thing that has always puzzled me about the "social transformation of American medicine" is the relatively silent role physicians have played. Anyone looking at the history of medicine 1940-1970 would have imagined that the medical profession was loud in defense of its own (supposed) interests and would not allow any other hands to be in control. I have noted how (for example) the EHR has deteriorated into a tool for billing, and away from what its pioneers intended it to be, with hardly a squawk from physicians as a group. The simplest answer I suppose is that physicians simply saw these developments as ways of increasing their own incomes and awoke too late. It is heartening that groups like the American College of Physicians are finally speaking up in favor of single payer.*

- Medical graduate in 1976 now completing 40 years' practice as a gastroenterologist in Connecticut, including 30 years in solo independent practice and 10 years employed by a hospital system:

> *There are almost no independent practitioners in my medical community at this time. All have signed on with the hospital for one reason or another. I could see this coming ten years ago; that virtually all of the physicians who had referred patients to me for the previous twenty years were not going to continue their referrals unless I was in their system, so I joined. Otherwise I would be sitting on my hands.*
>
> *I have lost control over every aspect of medical care except for what goes on in the examination room. Insurance companies, my employer, and pharmacy benefit managers are now in control of everything else.*

In addition, the culture in medicine and medical practice today has markedly changed, with most incoming medical graduates and other health professionals now wanting a well-paying job and a comfortable life style without too much night call.

2. Further Reasons to be Pessimistic about Health Care Reform

I believe that it is harder today than 20 years ago to get single-payer Medicare for All (NHI) moving forward and enacted, for these reasons:

- The alliance of deep pocketed corporate stakeholders invested in the status quo gets stronger all the time.

- Health care is highly profitable to corporate giants, their shareholders and Wall Street investors; health care fraud is also now estimated to account for $350 billion a year [6].
- The powerful U.S. Chamber of Commerce is resisting most efforts to rein in corporate crime. According to a research report by *Public Citizen*, its 111 members (the Chamber does not disclose its membership) represent big corporations ranging from the largest banks and oil-gas companies to high tech monopolists such as Amazon, Facebook and Google. The U.S. Chamber lobbies hard against enforcement by the Federal Trade Commission (FTC) while the annual cost of corporate and white-collar crime is estimated at between $300 and $800 billion a year [7].
- The press appears not to give credit for Biden's accomplishments, such as strong jobs reports, low unemployment, rebound of economy while focusing on inflation at highest level since 1981 without mentioning corporate profits at a 70-year high [8, 9].
- The two major political parties are more polarized than ever, with bipartisanship at an all-time low. While the Democrats advocate for more progressive legislation, taxing the rich, and a larger role of government, the Republicans protect the corporations as they argue for "fiscal responsibility" and a limited role of government [10].
- The battle over the cost and content of Biden's *Build Back Better* plan has taken over our politics and made this a more difficult time to get single-payer NHI heard with a high priority.
- The Biden administration doesn't yet understand the gravity of health care dysfunction, how all incremental reform attempts have failed, including the ACA, and is supportive of further privatization of Medicare.
- We have a McConnell and GOP-controlled Senate that blocks legislation, even a Voting Rights Act, with elimination of the filibuster still beyond reach.
- Citizens United remains a barrier to reform, as evidenced by the massive increase of federal campaign contributions from billionaires from 2010, when it was passed, to 2020 [11]. (Figure 14.1.)
- A 2020 report by Open Secrets, *More Money, Less Transparency: A Decade Under Citizens United*, found that election-related spending from non-party independent groups ballooned to $4.5 billion between 2010 and 2020, having been just $750 million in the preceding

decade. Figure 14.2 shows that just a very few of the wealthiest billionaires gave far more to federal campaigns than all other billionaires from 2000 to 2020 [12]. Is this what we want in our supposed democracy for the people?

- The power of money and wealth in the Congress raises still another concern about what happens with any legislative proposal that could rein in corporate abuses and revenues through Wall Street. Going into the 2020 elections, as one example, 93 of the 100 Senate members and 405 of the 435 House members were in the top 10 percent of wealth in the country. That raises the question whether they can understand and relate to the needs of ordinary Americans whom they represent [13].

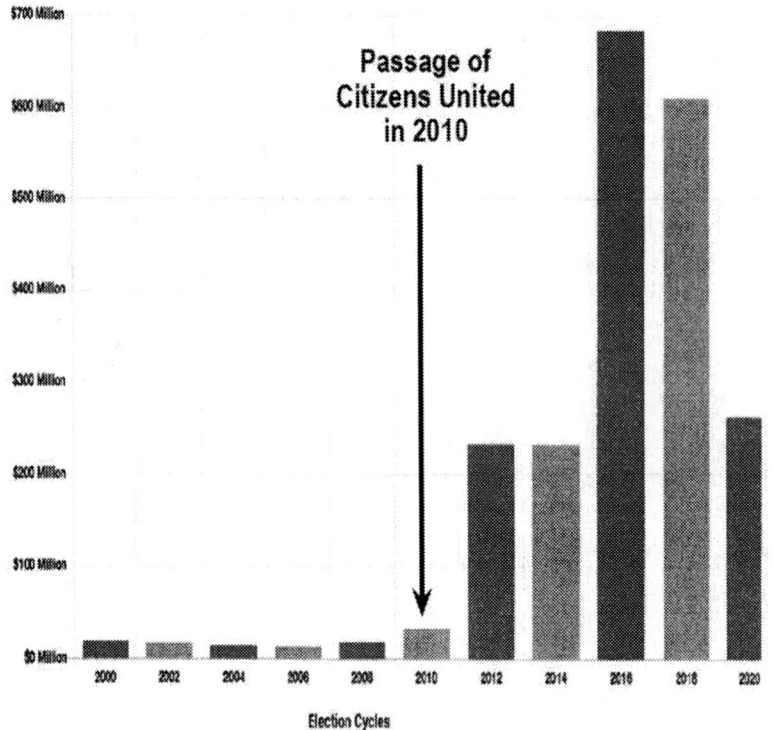

Source: Americans for Tax Fairness and the Institute for Policy Studies Inequality Program.

Figure 14.1. Federal campaign contributions from billionaires, 2000-2019.

"Free Market" Profiteering vs. Not-for-Profit Patient Care

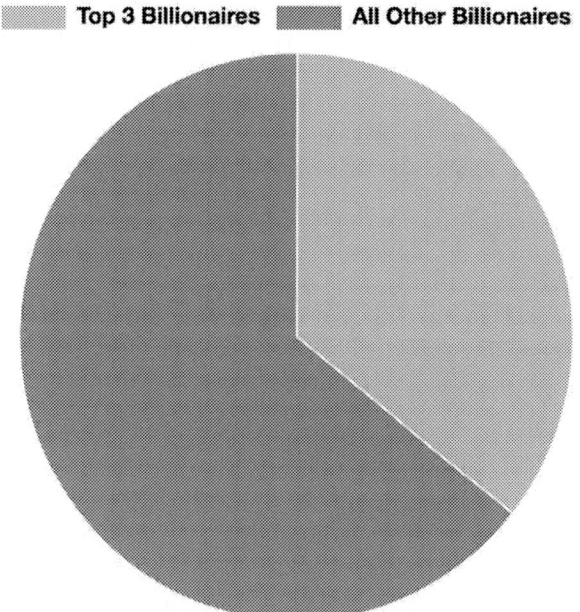

The top 3 billionaire contributors account for nearly 36%, or $763 million, of all billionaire contributions during the 1990 to 2020 election cycles.

The top 20 billionaire contributors account for nearly 62%, or $1.3 billion, of all billionaire contributions during the 1990 to 2020 election cycles.

Source: Billionaires by the numbers. Billionaires political influence. *Americans for Tax Fairness*, 2020.

Figure 14.2. Top 3 federal campaign contributors vs. all other billionaire contributors, 2000-2020.

- The power and money of lobbyists, plus the revolving door between industry, government, and K Street, remains a barrier to reform, as illustrated by what happened before passage of the 21st Century Cures Act in 2016. The bill added $6.3 billion to the search for new therapies for cancer and Alzheimer's disease as well as ways to advance genomics-based "precision medicine." Big PhRMA funded most of the 1,300 lobbyists working for the bill, and in return the final bill weakened the quality of scientific evidence required to demonstrate the safety and efficacy of new drugs and medical devices [14].

3. Reasons for Guarded Optimism about Future Health Care Reform

1. The need for universal coverage under single-payer Medicare for All, despite the challenges, becomes ever more urgent with each passing year than in the past, for these reasons:
   - The current system is falling apart and is unsustainable in its present form; as it becomes even more unaffordable, with worse access and quality, public and political pressure will grow for reform.
   - Public support for health care reform is already strong; the analysis of a massive data set mentioned in the opening paragraph found— that 87 percent of Americans favor congressional action to lower the cost of prescription drugs, that 79 percent are dissatisfied with the cost of their health care, and that 68 percent favor public health insurance over commercial insurance [15].
   - Health care is already unaffordable for many Americans, with the average family of four paying $28,256 a year for health insurance and care [16]; the median average annual household income for families in that year was $67,463.
   - 42 percent of patients with cancer age 50 or older have depleted their life savings in two years [17].
   - The Affordable Care Act has completely failed to contain costs and prices of health care.
   - Income inequality is more extreme today, with increasing numbers of Americans living in poverty.
   - The safety net is in tatters, while Medicaid coverage is winding down as the COVID pandemic eases [18], and as many Americans are dying preventable deaths.
   - Employer-sponsored insurance is more unreliable as people change jobs more frequently and often lose their insurance with their next job.
   - Private insurance is more restrictive with higher deductibles and co-pays, changing networks, and limited drug formularies, and then exiting markets that are not sufficiently lucrative [19].

2. Other reasons for potential optimism:
   - A new bill, Stop Corporate Capture Act (H.R. 6107) was introduced in December 2021 by Rep. Pramila Jayapal (D-WA), chair of the Congressional Progressive Caucus, with the goal to reduce corporate domination and increase the influence of consumers, workers, and ordinary Americans. If enacted, it would roll back corporate influence on the rulemaking process, remove industry-backed bottlenecks that thwart public protections, and increase transparency [20].
   - A recent poll by Data for Progress and the Revolving Door Project found that 70 percent of Republicans, Democrats and Independents all want the Biden administration to do more to fight corporate crime [21]. Another new Ipsos/PhRMA poll found that 92 percent of Democrats and 84 percent of Republicans strongly support cracking down on health insurance practices that make it harder for people to get the care that they need. Voters overwhelmingly support policies that would lower out-of-pocket costs and bring greater transparency to the health insurance system [22].
   - Tax reform is getting underway with President Biden's recent unveiling of a 20 percent minimum tax rate on all American households worth more than $100 million—now known as the "billionaire's tax." It would force the top 10 billionaires alone to pay $215 billion over the next decade, leading Americans for Tax Fairness to this comment:

Right now in America, 704 billionaires own more wealth than 65 million households. We can build an economy that works for the rest of us, but we need billionaires to pay their fair share [23].

   That kind of tax reform would be a big step forward, since 55 large corporations made $40 billion in U.S. profits in 2021 and paid no federal income tax [24].
   - Further, international crises such as the current battle between Russia and the West over Ukraine, ramp up the importance of health care reform.

4. Corporate Power vs. The Public Interest: Which Will Prevail?

This is still an open question, which must be answered in a way that places patients first. Physicians and other health professionals can be counted on to strongly advocate for the value of caring and universal coverage. Answering this question will test our democracy to its limits since it will require winning over the power and money of the medical-industrial complex.

As discussed in Chapter 12, there are four major reform alternatives for debate when health care reform can be on the front burner again in a Congress now fully engaged with the economy, the pandemic, and the international implications of the war in Ukraine. The first three are incremental GOP proposals—building on the ACA, some variant of a public option, and privatized Medicare Advantage for All. None would ever contain prices and costs of health care or achieve universal coverage. All three would continue to serve corporate interests in the medical-industrial complex at the expense of patients, families and taxpayers. The fourth proposal, single payer Medicare for All, would establish a system of universal coverage through national health insurance.

Separating health care from the strangle-hold of corporate interests is, of course, the single largest impediment to reform. If the U.S. were to get past this by setting up a transitional National Health Service (NHS) on the way to Medicare for All and NHI, we could look to Scotland for a success story. NHS Scotland was established in 1950 and is still going strong in providing universal coverage. The majority of its costs are paid through taxation, including all prescriptions filled in Scotland. It is the biggest employer in the country, and has a strong system of primary care based on general practice. It has led the world in new pioneering achievements, including the first practical ultrasound machines without radiation risks (1958), the first custom built organ transplantation centre (1968), and the world's first clinical service for MRI (1980). Private health insurance is also available, but is not mainstream [25].

These words by John Nichols, Washington correspondent for *The Nation* and author of the 2022 book, *Coronavirus Criminals and Pandemic Profiteers: Accountability for Those Who Caused the Crisis*, as well as *The Fight for the Soul of the Democratic Party*, *The Genius of Impeachment*, and *The "S" Word*, brings us this helpful observation:

It is not enough to defeat an insurrectionist president while his minions continue to run roughshod in the Senate. It is not enough to trade a Donald Trump in 2020 for a Trump 2.0 in 2024. It is not enough to expose a profiteering pharmaceutical company and let it continue to profiteer, or to note that billionaires got richer during the pandemic and then sit back and watch them become trillionaires [26].

Fast forward to 2040 and what kind of health care can we expect in the U.S.? It all depends, of course, on how effective the reform process, challenging at best, has been. Table 14.1 summarizes what we can expect of the outcome, whether or not the corporate octopus hold on health care persists or not.

Table 14.1. Alternative scenarios for 2040

FOR-PROFIT CORPORATE "SYSTEM" vs.	NOT-FOR-PROFIT NHS WITH NHI
Health care unaffordable	Affordable for patients and taxpayers
Worse access and quality of care	Improved access and quality
Increased fragmentation	Increased continuity of care
Primary care in tatters	Strengthened primary care
Poor distribution of care	Improved distribution to rural and underserved areas
Increased bureaucracy and waste	Simplified administration
Public and professional dissatisfaction	Strong public and professional satisfaction
Inefficient with high administrative overhead	Efficient, low administrative overhead
Poor system performance	Improved system performance
Unsustainable non-system	Sustainable rebuilt system

Rebuilding health care in this country on an ethic of service, and separating it from its present exploitation by mega-merged corporations motivated by maximizing revenues, will call for re-establishing a moral code and revived leadership from the medical profession and other health professions. Dr. Don Berwick, whom we met in Chapter 12, observes:

> *When the fabric of communities upon which health depends is torn, then healers are called to mend it. The moral law within us insists so. Improving the social determinants of health will be brought at last to a boil only by the heat of the moral determinants of health* [27].

We can also be guided by this prescient observation by a leading medical ethicist who understood what was happening in 1990:

> *Medicine is at heart a moral enterprise and those who practice it are de facto members of a moral community. We can accept or repudiate that fact, but we cannot ignore it or absolve ourselves of the moral consequences of our choice. We are not a guild, business, trade union, or a political party. If the care of the sick is increasingly treated as a commodity, an investment opportunity, a bureaucrat's power trip, or a political trading chip; the profession bears part of the responsibility* [28].
>
> —Edmund Pellegrino, M.D., physician, ethicist, moral philosopher, founder and director for many years of Georgetown University's Center for the Advanced Study of Ethics.

The Hastings Center Report on the Goals of Medicine in 1996 brought us this further helpful observation:

> *Everything can be bought and sold, turned into a commodity. But some goods, values, and institutions can too easily be corrupted by commodification. Health is a vital human good, and medicine a basic way of promoting it. Commercializing them, even for the sake of choice or efficiency, runs a potent risk of subverting them. The integrity of medicine is at stake. An excessive and unbalanced commercialization and privatization of medicine is a dire threat to the very goals of medicine* [29].

Uwe Reinhardt, Ph.D., Professor of Political Economy and Public Affairs at Princeton University, where he taught for almost 50 years, analyzed health systems around the world and was a supporter of single payer—but not in the U.S. In his excellent 2019 book, *Priced Out: The Economic and Ethical Costs of American Health Care*, he had these overriding reservations:

> *I have not advocated the single payer model here because our government is too corrupt . . . The key to a single payer system is that the*

government sets prices. Usually, it empowers boards of independent experts who set those prices low . . . In the United States, health industry interests have so much sway over Congress that the prices would end up being set by health-care interests. When you go to Taiwan or Canada, the kind of lobbying we have here is illegal there [30].

Equity and justice in health care for all Americans must remain the guiding lodestar throughout the process of reforming U.S. health care. We will need a larger role of government to oversee and implement reform, during which these words by Thomas Jefferson provide further guidance:

The care of human life and happiness, and not their destruction, is the first and only legitimate object of good government.

—In an address to the Republican Citizens of Washington County, Maryland in 1809

Many of us here today will not live to see what medicine and health care will be like in this country in 2040, but we hope that the Phoenix will have risen from ashes of our present failing health care non-system. (Figure 14.3) Only time will tell, and the clock is ticking . . .

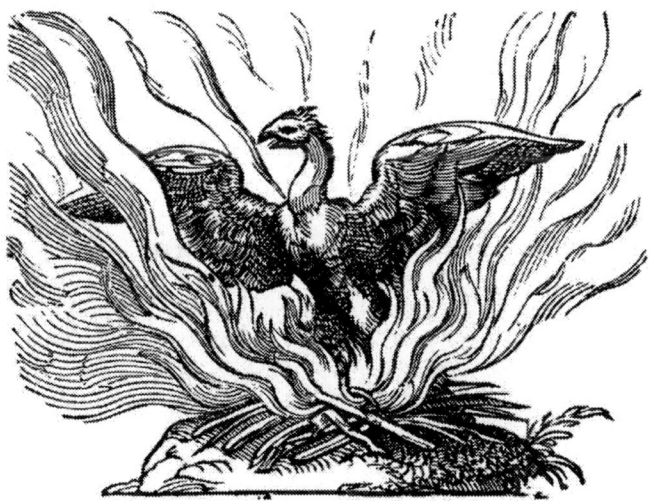

Phoenix rising from the Ashes, wood engraving from Latin edition of Pliny, Frankfort, 1602.

Figure 14.3. Phoenix rising from the ashes.

References

[1] Gilens, M, Page, B. Testing theories of American politics: Elites, interest groups, and average citizens. *Perspectives on Politics* 12 (3): 564-581, 2014.
[2] Swenson, P. House of Medicine for Rent. *Medscape Internal Medicine*, March 19, 2022.
[3] Ibid # 2.
[4] Lundberg, GD. Severed Trust: Why American Medicine Hasn't Been Fixed. New York. Basic Books, 2000, pp. 271, 289.
[5] Geyman, JP. The business "ethic" vs. service ethic in U.S. health care: Which will prevail? *The Pharos,* 2022.
[6] Estimate by Professor Malcolm Sparrow; personal communication from Ralph Nader, January 30, 2021.
[7] Cazemiro, A. U.S. Chamber of Commerce's war against FTC enforcement. *Public Citizen News*, March/April 2022, 9-10.
[8] Boehlert, E. Why is the press rooting against Biden? *The Progressive Populist*, May 1, 2022, p. 16.
[9] Reich, R. The highest inflation in 40 years. Americans need to know why. *Inequality Media*, April 20, 2022.
[10] Hartmann, T. What do Democrats and Republicans actually believe in 2022? That should decide the midterms. *The Progressive Populist*, February 15, 2022, p. 13.
[11] Clemente, F. Billionaires by the numbers. *Americans for Tax Fairness & The Institute for Policy Studies Inequality Program*, July 15, 2020.
[12] Evers-Hillstrom, K, Weber, D, Massoglia, A et al. More money, less transparency: A decade under Citizen United, *Open Secrets*, January 14, 2020.
[13] Abramson, J. *Sickening: How Big PhRMA Broke American Health Care and How We Can Repair It.* New York. HarperCollins Publishers, 2022, pp. 199-200.
[14] Billionaires by the numbers. Billionaires political influence. *Americans for Tax Fairness*, 2020.
[15] Ibid # 1.
[16] Milliman Medical Index, 2021.
[17] Haefner, M. Two years after cancer diagnosis, 42% of patients age 50 or older have depleted their life savings. National Institute of Aging, as reported by *Becker's Hospital CFO Report*, October 24, 2018.
[18] Brooks Tricia, Allexa Gardner, Aubrianna Osorio, Jennifer Tolbert , Bradley Corallo, Meghana Ammula, and Sophia Moreno. Medicaid and CHIP eligibility and enrollment policies as of January 2022: Findings from a 50-state survey. *Kaiser Family Foundation*, March 16, 2022.
[19] Tracer, Z, Darie, T. More than 1 million in Obamacare lose plans as insurers quit. *Bloomberg News*, October 14, 2016.
[20] Rosen, D. Bill to end corporate capture of the regulatory process gains support. *Public Citizen News*, March/April 2002, 7.
[21] Claypool, R. The time for corporate accountability is now. *Public Citizen News*, March/April 2002, 10, 15.

[22] McCanne, D. Comment on PhRMA attacks insurers and new Ipsos poll shows Americans are frustrated with abusive insurance practices that exacerbate access and affordability. *Health Justice Monitor*, March 28, 2022.
[23] Queally, J. Biden tax plan would force top 10 billionaires alone to pay $215 billion over next decade. *Common Dreams*, March 27, 2022.
[24] Nader, R. In the Public Interest. Going for tax reform big time. *The Progressive Populist*, April 15, 2022, p. 19.
[25] Healthcare in Scotland (https://www.scotland.org).
[26] Nichols, J. *Coronavirus Criminals and Pandemic Profiteers: Accountability for Those Who Caused the Crisis*, New York. *Verso*, 2022, p. 268.
[27] Berwick, D. The moral determinants of health. *JAMA* 324 (3): 226, 2020.
[28] Pellegrino, ED. The medical profession as a moral community. Bulletin. *Bull NY Acad Med* 66 (3): 222, 1990.
[29] Project Report. *The Goals of Medicine: Setting New Priorities*. Special Supplement. *Hastings Center Report*, November-December 1996: S-20-21.
[30] Reinhardt, UE. *Priced Out: The Economic and Ethical Costs of American Health Care.* Princeton, NJ. *Princeton University Press*, 2019, pp. 152-153.

About the Author

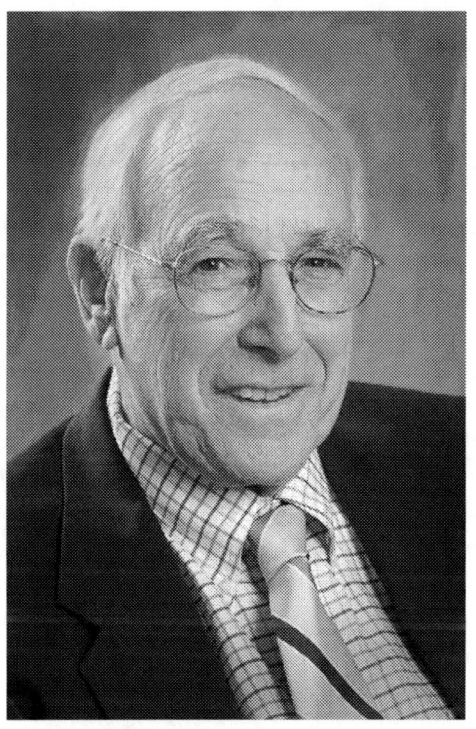

John Geyman, MD is Professor Emeritus of Family Medicine at the University of Washington School of Medicine in Seattle, where he served as Chairman of the Department of Family Medicine from 1976 to 1990. As a family physician with over 21 years in academic medicine, he also practiced in rural communities for 13 years. He was the founding editor of *The Journal of Family Practice* (1973 to 1990) and the editor of *The Journal of the American Board of Family Medicine* from 1990 to 2003. Since 1990 he has been involved with research and writing on health policy and health care reform.

His most recent books were: *Are We the UNITED States of America? Can We Hold Together as One Country?* (2022), *Transformation of U.S. Health Care 1960-2020: One Family Physician's Journey* (2022), *America's Mighty Medical-Industrial Complex: Negative Impacts and Positive Solutions* (2021), and *Profiteering, Corruption and Fraud in U.S. Health Care* (2020).

Earlier books included: *Long Term Care In America: The Crisis All Of Us Will Face In Our Lifetimes* (2020), *Struggling and Dying After Trumpcare* (2019), *TrumpCare: Lies, Broken Promises, How It Is Failing, and What Should Be Done?* (2018), *Crisis in U.S. Health Care: Corporate Power vs. the Common Good* (2017), *The Human Face of ObamaCare: Promises vs. Reality and What Comes Next* (2016), *How Obamacare Is Unsustainable: Why We Need a Single-Payer Solution For All Americans* (2015), *Health Care Wars: How Market Ideology and Corporate Power Are Killing Americans* (2012), *Souls On a Walk: An Enduring Love Story Unbroken by Alzheimer's* (2012), *Breaking Point: How the Primary Care Crisis Threatens the Lives of Americans* (2011), *Hijacked: The Road to Single Payer in the Aftermath of Stolen Health Care Reform* (2010), *The Cancer Generation: Baby Boomers Facing a Perfect Storm* (2009), *Do Not Resuscitate: Why the Health Insurance Industry Is Dying* (2008), *The Corrosion of Medicine: Can the Profession Reclaim Its Moral Legacy* (2008), *Shredding the Social Contract: The Privatization of Medicare* (2006), *Falling Through the Safety Net: Americans Without Health Insurance* (2005), T*he Corporate Transformation of Health Care: Can the Public Interest Still Be Served?* (2004), *Health Care in America: Can Our Ailing System Be Healed?* (2002), and *The Modern Family Doctor and Changing Medical Practice* (1971).

John has also published five pamphlets following the approach of Thomas Paine in 1775-1776: *Common Sense About Health Care Reform in America* (2017), *Common Sense: U.S. Health Care at a Crossroads in the 2018 Congress* (2018), *Common Sense: The Case For and Against Medicare For All. Leading Issue in the 2020 Elections* (2019), *Common Sense: Medicare For All: Foundation for a 'New Normal' In U.S. Health Care* (2020), and *Common Sense: Medicare For All: What Will It Mean For Me?* (2021)

He also served as the president of Physicians for a National Health Program from 2005 to 2007, and is a member of the National Academy of Medicine.

Email: jgeyman@uw.edu

Index

A

Aduhelm, 28, 48
Affordable Care Act (ACA), 18, 19, 20, 22, 49, 53, 61, 93, 94, 95, 111, 118, 125, 126, 129, 130, 133, 149, 152, 154
   bureaucracy and administrative waste, 130, 136
American Antitrust Institute, 105, 108
American Hospital Association (AHA), 110, 117, 131
American Medical Association (AMA), 69, 106, 110, 117, 120, 136, 146
Americans for Tax Fairness, 150, 151, 153, 158
Arrow, K., 10, 12

B

Bauchner, H., 136, 142
Baucus, M., 118, 121
Being Mortal: Medicine and What Matters in the End (Gawande, A.), 95
Benchmarks for Fairness for Health Care Reform (Light, D.), 73
Berwick, D., 121, 125, 132, 155, 159
Blue Cross and Blue Shield, 3, 23

C

Center for Medicare and Medicaid Innovation, 19, 118
Center for Studying Health System Change, 10
Churchill, W., 114
Citizens United, 149

Clinical Ethics: A Practical Approach to Clinical Decisions in Clinical Medicine (Jonsen, A.), 5
Committee on the Costs of Medical Care, 3
Commonwealth Fund, 57, 58, 59, 60, 63, 65, 79, 97, 132
   cross national research in 11 advanced countries, 57, 58, 61
Coronavirus Criminals and Pandemic Profiteers: Accountability for Those Who Caused the Crisis (Nichols, J.), 154, 159
corporate power vs public interest, 85
corporatization, 146
corruption, xiv, 41, 99
cost-effectiveness, 29, 32, 126, 136
cost-effectiveness analysis, 29, 32, 126
COVID-19
   pandemic
      international comparisons, 64, 77
      lessons for future pandemics, 77, 85
      performance of U. S. health care, 79
COVID-19 pandemic, 22, 73, 77
Cronkite, W., 55
culture of, 3, 4

D

Deadly Spin: An Insurance Company Insider Speaks Out on How Corporate PR Is Killing Health Care and Deceiving Americans (Potter, W.), 22
Deaths of Despair and the Future of Capitalism (Deaton and Case), 49
Deaton, A., 67
DeSalvo, K., 64, 66
Disorder: A History of Reform, Reaction, and Money in American Medicine (Swenson, P.), 146

Index

disparities, 58, 62, 64, 65, 67, 70, 71, 74, 75, 76, 84, 126, 138

E

Eisenhower, D., 9
electronic health records, 5
   as billing instrument, 5
Everything for Sale and the End of Laissez-Faire (Kuttner, R.), 101, 135

F

Financial Times, 85, 86, 87
Fisher, E., 13, 30, 31, 33, 42, 132
for a National Health Program, v, 97, 100, 108, 140, 141, 162
Fowler, E., 117, 121
fraud, xiv, 40, 43, 53, 64, 84, 99, 149
   of billing practices, 40
Friedman, G., 87, 94, 97, 139, 142
Friedson, E., 100, 107

G

Gaffney, A., 24, 97, 140, 143
Giroux, H. A., 109, 120
Goldman, D., 66, 106, 108
Goliath: The 100-Year War between Monopoly Power and Democracy (Stoller, M.), 99, 107

H

Hastings Bioethics Research Institute, 46
health care, v, ix, xi, xii, xiii, xiv, 3, 4, 5, 6, 7, 8, 9, 10, 11, 12, 13, 15, 16, 18, 23, 25, 27, 28, 29, 30, 31, 32, 35, 36, 37, 38, 40, 41, 42, 43, 45, 46, 47, 48, 49, 51, 52, 53, 54, 55, 57, 58, 59, 60, 61, 62, 63, 64, 65, 67, 69, 73, 74, 75, 76, 77, 79, 80, 84, 85, 86, 87, 90, 91, 93, 94, 95, 96, 97, 99, 101, 102, 104, 105, 106, 107, 108, 109, 112, 113, 114, 115, 116, 117, 119, 120, 123, 125, 126, 127, 128, 129, 131, 132, 133, 135, 136, 138, 140, 141, 142, 143, 145, 146, 147, 149, 152, 153, 154, 155, 157, 158, 161
access to, xiii, 10, 21, 35, 60, 61, 83, 126, 130
as human right, 52, 69, 73, 136
barriers to, xiii, 6, 10, 57, 60, 61, 74
bureaucracy of, 18, 93, 128, 130, 136
commodification of, 46, 107, 109, 156
corporatization of, 146
costs of, xi, xiii, 3, 8, 9, 10, 13, 15, 16, 18, 20, 23, 24, 25, 27, 28, 29, 30, 32, 33, 35, 36, 37, 42, 43, 49, 57, 61, 62, 65, 71, 74, 80, 81, 86, 87, 89, 90, 91, 93, 94, 96, 97, 102, 106, 109, 117, 126, 127, 128, 129, 130, 137, 138, 139, 142, 152, 153, 154
disparities and, 58, 62, 64, 65, 67, 70, 71, 74, 75, 76, 84, 126, 138
equity of, 58
financing of, ix, 15, 17, 23, 41, 60, 64, 74, 85, 89, 91, 96, 109, 110, 114, 119, 136, 137, 138, 139, 141
and value-based payments, 118
hospitalists and, 5
inequities of, 62, 64, 67, 69, 70, 71, 73, 74, 80, 84, 129, 138
investor-owned vs. not-for-profit, xiii, 4, 10, 13, 19, 37, 42, 61, 99, 101
managed care, 18, 19, 24, 37, 48, 72, 76, 90, 94, 97, 100, 126, 132
quality of, xiii, 10, 13, 22, 30, 37, 42, 48, 49, 50, 54, 57, 61, 71, 73, 74, 102, 104, 106, 117, 126, 127, 128, 131, 132, 138, 140, 141, 151, 152
racism and, 64, 67, 69, 72, 73, 74, 75, 76, 85
reform and, ix, xii, xiv, 6, 12, 41, 52, 64, 73, 85, 96, 106, 107, 108, 109, 111, 112, 113, 114, 115, 117, 119, 120, 123, 125, 127, 130, 131, 132, 135, 136, 138, 140, 141, 142, 145, 147, 149, 151, 152, 153, 154, 155, 157, 159, 161

reform and lessons from failed attempts, 109
safety net and, 10, 80, 126, 152
unaffordability of, 126, 127
universal coverage for, 23, 60, 61, 64, 73, 85, 109, 110, 115, 119, 129, 131, 139, 152, 154
health insurance, v, ix, xii, 15, 16, 20, 22, 23, 24, 25, 28, 32, 43, 49, 57, 61, 64, 65, 66, 71, 79, 80, 89, 90, 91, 92, 95, 97, 110, 112, 115, 116, 120, 125, 129, 135, 137, 138, 139, 142, 146, 147, 152, 153, 154
benefits of, 107
conventional theory of, 90
cost sharing and, 22, 71, 90, 91, 104, 127, 130, 137
denial of services, 18, 22
employer-sponsored, 9, 16, 22, 24, 71, 79, 90, 91, 93, 97, 116, 142
history of, 67, 90, 99
National Health Service and, 94, 97, 141, 142, 154
pre-authorization and, 92, 139
unaffordable costs and, xiii, 6, 10, 30
uninsured, 11, 22, 57, 126, 130, 132, 137, 141
universal coverage and, 23, 60, 73
health insurers, 20, 24, 38, 53, 87, 90, 91, 93, 94, 97, 118, 120, 126, 137
bureaucracy of, 18, 93, 128, 130, 136
profiteering by, xiii, 5, 10, 15, 28, 30, 35, 37, 38, 39, 41, 49, 52, 81, 84, 85, 99, 118, 126, 127, 129, 131, 135, 145, 155
volatility of, 92, 95, 106
Hightower, J., 65, 102, 107
Himmelstein, D.U., 7, 13, 33, 42, 100, 107, 132, 133, 141, 143
Hippocratic oath, 46, 49, 53
Hope or Hype: The Obsession with Medical Advances and the High Cost of False Promises (Deyo, R. and Patrick, D.), 25, 33
hospices, 13, 40, 42, 101

Hughes, R., 57, 65

I

Institute for Policy Studies, 71, 75, 150, 158
Institute of Medicine, 64, 66

J

Jefferson, T., 157

K

Kahn, J., 12
Kinser, K., 17
Kristof, N., 55, 68, 75
Kuttner, R., 101, 107, 123, 135, 142

L

License to Steal: How Fraud Bleeds America's Health Care System (Sparrow, M.), 40, 43, 53
Light, D., 73, 76, 121
Lown, B., 15, 23, 101, 107
Ludmerer, K., 100, 107
Lundberg, G., 146, 158

M

McConnell, M., 117, 149
Medicaid, xi, 3, 6, 19, 20, 21, 24, 37, 42, 48, 62, 69, 72, 75, 76, 80, 90, 92, 93, 94, 97, 118, 125, 128, 129, 130, 132, 138, 152, 158
and overpayments, 19, 22, 37, 48, 94, 131, 138
expansion of, 79
medical devices, 29, 33, 139, 151
and FDA approval, 29
medical practice
administrators, 7
after-hours care, 5, 63
medical technology, xi, 26, 32

evaluation and approval of, 29
levels of, 29, 30
medical-industrial complex, 1, 3, 4, 9, 10, 11, 15, 25, 32, 36, 46, 52, 73, 81, 112, 135, 136, 154
   Adverse impacts of, 10
   corporate ownership in, 3, 4, 7, 9
Medicare, xi, xii, 3, 6, 13, 18, 19, 20, 21, 22, 23, 24, 29, 33, 37, 38, 40, 42, 43, 48, 53, 65, 69, 73, 82, 87, 90, 92, 93, 94, 95, 97, 98, 104, 115, 116, 117, 118, 119, 120, 121, 125, 127, 128, 130, 131, 132, 133, 137, 138, 139, 140, 141, 142, 143, 146, 147, 148, 149, 152, 154, 162
   and overpayments, 19, 22, 37, 48, 94, 131, 138
   for All, 22, 23, 42, 73, 97, 115, 116, 117, 119, 120, 130, 132, 133, 137, 138, 140, 141, 142, 148, 152, 154
   for some, 130
   privatized vs. public, ix, 19
   The Case for Medicare for All (Friedman, G.), 94, 139, 142
Medicare Advantage, 19, 21, 22, 24, 48, 94, 95, 97, 98, 118, 121, 130, 132, 133, 137, 154
   for All, 22, 130, 133, 154
Milliman Medical Index, xi, 8, 12, 97, 158
More Money, Less Transparency: A Decade Under Citizens United (Open Secrets), 149
   and expansion of corporate power, 150
Moyers, Bill, 55, 118, 121

N

Nader, R., v, 43, 119, 120, 121, 158, 159
National Medical Association, 69, 73

O

Oberlander, J., 78, 86

P

Pellegrino, E., 45, 52, 156, 159
Petris Center at the University of California Berkeley, 105
Pew Research Center, 67, 71
Phillips, B., 47, 53
Physicians, v, 5, 15, 23, 38, 46, 47, 53, 97, 100, 106, 108, 140, 141, 148, 154, 162
   and independent practice, 50, 148
   burnout, 6, 51, 106
   clinical autonomy of, xiii, 5, 50, 106
   early retirements, 6, 106
   EHR/desk work, 6
   suicide, 6
Politics after Hope: Obama and the Crisis of Youth, Race and Democracy (Henry A. Giroux, H. A.), 109
Potter, W., 22, 24, 43, 87, 97, 115, 117, 120
Priced Out: The Economic and Ethical Costs of American Health Care (Reinhardt, U.), 61, 65, 156, 159
private equity, 36, 37, 38, 40, 41, 43, 53, 99, 101, 102, 104, 105, 107, 108, 135, 141
   profiteering by, 37
   purchase of physicians' practices, 38, 48, 104
privatization of public programs, 4
   Medicaid, 18
   Medicare, 18
profiteering, xiii, 5, 10, 15, 28, 30, 35, 37, 38, 39, 41, 49, 52, 81, 84, 85, 99, 118, 126, 127, 129, 131, 135, 145, 155
   across the medical-industrial complex, 10, 21, 99
   hospitals, xiii, 3, 4, 13, 21, 30, 36, 37, 38, 41, 42, 43, 49, 53, 62, 63, 64, 65, 69, 80, 81, 87, 89, 90, 92, 96, 97, 101, 102, 104, 116, 117, 131, 137, 139, 141
   jails, 37, 42, 65
   pharmaceutical industry, 146
   private health insurers, 10

Index

between drug manufacturers and pharmacy benefit managers, 27
by direct contracting entities (DCEs), 19
by drug companies, 101
public health, 3, 35, 64, 74, 77, 78, 79, 85, 86, 95, 111, 136, 141, 152
underfunding of public health, 77

R

Reinhardt, U., 61, 65, 156, 159
Relman, A., 1, 45, 52
Roosevelt, Franklin Delano, 110, 112
Roosevelt, Teddy, 73, 110
Rosenthal, E., 35, 41

S

Severed Trust: Why American Medicine Hasn't Yet Been Fixed (Lundberg, G.), 147
Sickening: How Big PhRMA Broke American Health Care and How We Can Repair It (Abramson, J.), 145, 158
Sigerist, H., 89, 96
single payer national health insurance, 111, 112, 115
Song, Z., 43, 53, 105, 108
Stephens, G., 51, 54
Stevens, R., 51, 54
Stoller, M., 99, 107
System Error: Where Big Tech Went Wrong and How We Can Reboot (Reich, R, Sahami, M., Weinstein, J.M.), 31, 33

T

The American Health Empire: Power, Profits and Politics (Ehrenreich, B. and J.), 4, 12
The Intellectual Basis of Family Practice (Stephens, G.), 51
The Political Life of Medicare (Oberlander, J.), 78
The Social Transformation of American Medicine (Starr, P.), 4, 12, 120
The Truth about Drug Companies How They Deceive Us and What We Can Do About It (Angell, M.), 107
Thomas, L., 17, 29, 33, 68, 157, 162
Thurow, L., 128, 132
Twain, M., 25, 45, 52

W

Wall Street, viii, xiv, 4, 9, 12, 13, 17, 22, 23, 24, 25, 33, 42, 52, 53, 54, 65, 68, 72, 73, 75, 76, 86, 87, 90, 96, 97, 99, 101, 106, 107, 108, 120, 133, 135, 140, 141, 146, 149, 150
adverse impacts on physicians and other health professionals, 99
adverse impacts on physicians and other health professionals, 146
and corporate America, 4, 9, 101, 106, 141
and leveraged buyout industry, 99
and transformation of U. S. health care, 99
Welch, G., 30, 31, 33
Who Will Tell the People: The Betrayal of American Democracy (Greider, W.), 119
Woolhandler, S., 7, 13, 33, 42, 100, 107, 132, 133, 141, 143